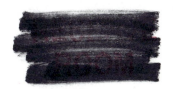

Critique, Resistance, and Action
Working Papers in the Politics
of Nursing

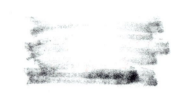

Critique, Resistance, and Action
Working Papers in the Politics of Nursing

Janice L. Thompson
David G. Allen
Lorraine Rodrigues-Fisher

Editors

National League for Nursing Press • New York
Pub. No. 14-2504

ISBN 0-88737-563-4

Library of Congress Cataloging-in-Publication Data

Critique, resistance, and action : working papers in the politics of
nursing / Janice L. Thompson, David G. Allen, Lorraine Rodrigues-
Fisher, editors.
        p.   cm.
    "Pub. no. 14-2504."
    Includes bibliographical references and index.
    ISBN 0-88737-563-4 : $38.95
    1. Nursing—Philosophy—Congresses.   2. Nursing—Political
aspects—Congresses.   3. Feminism—Congresses.   I. Allen, David,
1948–   . I. Thompson, Janice L. III. Rodrigues-Fisher,
Lorraine.
    [DNLM: 1. Nursing—congresses.   2. Nursing Theory—con-
gresses.   3. Women—congresses.   WY 86 C934]
RT84.5.C77   1992
810.73—dc20
DNLM/DLC
for Library of Congress   92-48677
                                                           CIP

Contents

Contributors   vii

Acknowledgements   ix

Introduction   xi

1. Feminism, Relativism, and the Philosophy of Science: An Overview   1
   David G. Allen

2. Identity Politics, Essentialism, and Constructions of "Home" in Nursing   21
   Janice L. Thompson

3. Race, Racism, and Health: Examining the "Natural Facts"   35
   Karen K. Maeda Allman

4. Eve's Legacy: An Analysis of Family Caregiving from a Feminist Perspective   53
   Sheila M. Bunting

v

5. Nursing and the Caring Metaphor: Gender and Political
   Influences on an Ethics of Care   69
   Esther H. Condon

6. A Feminist Critique of Jean Watson's Theory of Caring   85
   D. Patricia Gray

7. Reproductive Technology and Court Ordered Obstetrical
   Interventions: The Need for a Feminist Voice in Nursing   97
   Elizabeth I. Hagell

8. Is Woman Born or Made? Female Gender Identity in
   Women's Health   117
   Dorothy J. Henderson

9. Language and the Reification of Nursing Care   129
   Akemi Hiraki

10. The Drive for Professionalism in Nursing: A Reflection of
    Classism and Racism   137
    Sally O'Neill

11. A Critical Analysis of Professionalism in Nursing   149
    Beatrice B. Turkoski

12. Perceptions and Feelings of Nurses about Horizontal
    Violence as an Expression of Oppressed Group Behavior   167
    Lois Napier Skillings

Index   187

Contributors

David G. Allen, PhD, RN, FAAN, is Associate Professor and Chair, Department of Psychosocial Nursing, University of Washington, Seattle, WA.

Karen K. Maeda Allman, PhC, RN, is a doctoral candidate, School of Nursing, University of Washington, Seattle, WA.

Sheila M. Bunting, PhC, RN, is a doctoral candidate, Division of Nursing, Wayne State University, Detroit, MI.

Esther H. Condon, PhD, RN, is Associate Professor and Chairperson, Department of Graduate Nursing Education, Hampton University, Hampton, VA.

Lorraine Rodrigues-Fisher, EdD, RN, is Associate Professor and Director, Center for Continuing Nursing Education, Medical College of Ohio, Toledo, OH.

D. Patricia Gray, PhD, RN, is Associate Professor and Coordinator of Graduate Programs, School of Nursing, Georgia State University, Atlanta, GA

Elizabeth I. Hagell, MEd, RN, is Instructor, Department of Nursing, Red Deer College, Red Deer, Alberta, Canada.

Dorothy J. Henderson, MS, RN, is a doctoral student, School of Nursing, University of Michigan, Ann Arbor, MI.

Akemi Hiraki, EdD, MSN, RN, is Lecturer, Department of Nursing, San Francisco State University, San Francisco, CA.

Sally O'Neill, MN, RN, is Nurse Clinician, Swedish Hospital Medical Center, Washington, Seattle, WA.

Janice L. Thompson, PhD, RN, is Associate Professor, School of Nursing, University of Southern Maine, Portland, ME.

Beatrice B. Turkoski, PhD, RN, is Assistant Professor, School of Nursing, Kent State University, Kent, OH.

Lois Napier Skillings, MSN, RN, CEN, is Coordinator of Clinical Nursing Services, Mid Coast Hospital, and Private Consultant in Nursing Staff Development, Brunswick, ME.

Acknowledgements

The papers in this collection were originally presented at the second national conference on Critical and Feminist Perspectives in Nursing, February, 1991, in Toledo, Ohio. We gratefully acknowledge the assistance of staff members at the Center for Continuing Nursing Education, Medical College of Ohio. Their work in facilitating the conference and in retyping drafts of these manuscripts made this collection possible.

Neither the conferences nor the work they represent would be possible if we were not standing on the shoulders of women who labored to keep feminist discourses and feminist visions of nursing and society alive. We know this was a labor of love for them and often entailed significant personal and political sacrifices. We hope they would see the work of these conferences and this book as forwarding their visions.

We also wish to acknowledge and thank the many participants who have supported this series of conferences. It is their personal, political, and intellectual commitments that have made the conferences possible and have, in turn, advanced the work of nurses committed to feminist and critical perspectives.

Foremost among these participants is D. Patricia Gray. Her community-building skills and ever deepening vision of a possible world for nursing have been indispensable to the success and continuation of the conferences and have contributed to the strengthening of feminist voices in nursing.

We thank all these people and students, colleagues, friends, and partners who have nurtured the ideas that appear in this book and challenged us all to bring them into nursing in new and different ways.

Introduction

The very meaning of "home" changes with the experience of decolonization, of radicalization. At times home is nowhere. At times one knows only extreme estrangement and alienation. Then home is no longer just one place. It is locations. Home is that place which enables and promotes varied and everchanging perspectives, a place where one discovers new ways of seeing reality, frontiers of difference. One confronts and accepts dispersal and fragmentation as part of the construction of a new world order that reveals more fully where we are, who we can become, an order that does not demand forgetting. Our struggle is also a struggle of memory against forgetting (hooks, 1991, p. 148).

Several schools of thought inform the work contained in this collection. The papers were originally presented at the Second Annual Conference on Critical and Feminist Perspectives in Nursing, February 1991, in Toledo, Ohio. In this forum, nurses presented work informed by feminist scholarship, critical theory or critical hermeneutics, and postmodern thought. But each of these works begins from the situated concerns of practicing nurses. The collection of essays examines a broad range of issues and demonstrates the influence of feminism, postmodern critique, and critical theory as discourses that challenge the politics of gender, race/ethnicity, class, and sex in the social constructions of nursing. Together, the essays provide a broad critique of power relations in nursing.

In this collection of essays, nurses speak from many radicalized places about the construction of reality and about nurses' lived experiences in dominant culture. Nurses are "at home" in these critical essays, informed by many different theories, schools of thought, paradigms, or critical perspectives regarding the social world. As works in progress, the papers illustrate how one can be "at home" in nursing, situated within the community of nursing, while engaging in critique.

There have always been nurses who spoke from the standpoint of critique, who claimed the margin and identified with the struggles of other diverse people as a position of strength and personal authority. Today, that voice of critique in nursing continues. Indeed, it is part of a larger cultural landscape, a postmodern world that is informed by many critical discourses.

In this book, we see work that illustrates the organic process of "speaking differently." Contrary to *some* (Western) models of scientific work, this is not so much a mechanical, instrumental process of mastering a theory and applying it to nursing practice. Rather, it is learning to speak, think, see, and be in the world from those places that are elsewhere, other than the dominant, center, colonizing, hegemonic world order.

In the United States, there are many political and intellectual forces influencing critique in nursing. The cultural climate of the 1990s reflects growing contradictions in our social, economic, and political structures, and many persons detect that our systems are in transition. This transitional space is also informed now by several diverse intellectual traditions, which have emerged on the scene as discourses of critique or "suspicion" (Alexander, 1991). These are conversations which are informed both by intellectual and political practice, critical traditions which challenge the hegemony of the dominant world order.

In the United States, critical work has touched all academic disciplines, and it would be unusual if this work did not appear in nursing literature and practice (Thompson, 1987). Feminism, in its second wave, emerged in the United States primarily as a social and political movement during the 1960s. But it eventually took root as an academic field of study with the introduction of women's studies programs during the 1970s. During the 1980s, fields such as Asian or African studies were recognized as antecedents of new programs in cultural studies. In many "established" disciplines as well, boundaries have been blurred and borders crossed by strategies with names like "geneology" and "deconstruction."

We live then in a time of transition where once accepted categories of social meaning are breaking down (Flax, 1989). In this transitional space, critical work can take many forms. Whether we experience it in the form of "in your face politics" or in the form of clear, firm action to build identity and develop ties around common struggles, critique is never theory divorced from practice. It *is* practice; practical intervention in the social world. The papers presented here reflect this commitment and demonstrate the ways in which nurses, speaking from various situated places, are working to transform the practice of nursing and the contexts in which nurses and patients meet. In many ways, this collection illustrates the transitions that have been made in nursing scholarship over the last 20 years. Collectively, the papers show us a trace of the ways in which nurses have moved in and through the traditions of phenomenology, hermeneutics, and postmodern critique to describe, interpret, and deconstruct the practices of nursing. This trace is full of flux, disruption, and seams (periodically unraveled) that illustrate common struggles and different, situated knowledges in nursing.

The influence of phenomenology can be seen in several of the essays, although none will demonstrate the assumptions of a foundationalist phenomenology. These papers break from grounded theory or naturalistic phenomenology in that they do not accept the possibility of a bracketed description. Instead, all of the papers argue that descriptions of phenomena are situated within historical horizons, within contexts, and that the situatedness of phenomena and phenomenologist will include "unbracketable" details like gender, class, race, sexual orientation, and so on. The convergence of feminist scholarship and phenomenological commitments can be seen, for example, in Patty Gray's paper, "A Feminist Critique of Jean Watson's Theory of Caring," in Esther Condon's paper, "Nursing and the Caring Metaphor: Gender and Political Influences on an Ethics of Care," in Sheila Bunting's essay, "Eve's Legacy: An Analysis of Family Caregiving from a Feminist Perspective," and in Dorothy Henderson's paper, "Is Woman Born or Made? Female Gender Identity in Women's Health." In each of these works, the authors argue that descriptions of phenomena must take seriously the category of gender, accounting for the ways in which our experiences of phenomena are gendered. Here we see nurses speaking (as other phenomenologists have) about our lived experiences in the world as embodied experiences and noticing that our identity in these bodies is gendered. This phenomenological insight is relevant in transpersonal discussions of caring, in metaphors of care as an ethic, in sociohistorical accounts of caregiver burden and strain, and in phenomenological accounts of the developing self.

The papers also include clear evidence of how nursing scholarship has moved in and through hermeneutic traditions. Several authors illustrate a "linguistic turn," a commitment to notice language, not as neutral, transparent medium, but rather as historically situated text or discourse with ideological functions. Hermeneutic influences come through in a series of papers which critically examine professional discourse and the history of professionalization in nursing. Akemi Hiraki's "Language and the Reification of Nursing Care" and Beatrice Turkoski's "A Critical Analysis of Professionalism in Nursing" include reviews of contemporary interpretive theory and illustrate the use of interpretive theory to critique professionalism. Sally O'Neill and Lois Skillings extend this critical hermeneutic research that critiques nursing's history of professionalization, examining race and class struggles in nursing and the dynamics of oppressed group behavior among staff nurses.

In addition, the papers collected here also reflect an awareness of the postmodern landscape. This perspective is illustrated in the authors' musings as they notice silences and gaps in their own work and as they situate themselves, or identify themselves, within the body of their work. Nurses who write here have learned important insights from postmodern feminist critique, which focused, for example, on the silences and gaps in white feminist scholarship. Postmodern feminist critique pointed out that white feminists did not situate themselves or their ideas as they made universalizing claims about a woman-centered perspective and gender as category (Tong, 1989). These insights are reflected in this collection in the recognition that lived experience and identities are multiple and that an individual's sense of self is determined by crisscrossing identities, multiple social roles, and interests which are split depending on gender, race, ethnicity, class, sexual orientation, age, and so on.

A postmodern critique in nursing also notices the ways in which discourses (e.g., white feminist scholarship) function as regimes of power, where knowledge and power interact to normalize or legitimate specific interests. Karen Maeda Allman's "Race, Racism and Health: Examining the Natural Facts," draws on the postmodern work of Michel Foucault and Donna Haraway. This paper specifically examines recent constructions of race in health literature and explores the ways in which nursing and medical discourse function to construct "the body" as a site of power and operations. Sally O'Neill's "The Drive for Professionalism in Nursing" also examines ways in which the constructions of white nurses functioned historically in the interaction between white and African-American nurses. And Elizabeth Hagell's "Reproductive Technology and Court Ordered Obstetrical Interventions" reviews contemporary nursing literature and locates a silence or an absence of any critical or feminist perspective in nursing related to reproductive care.

The first two chapters, by Allen and Thompson, address themes that are either picked up by or form the background for several others. Thompson's

"Identity Politics, Essentialism and Constructions of 'Home' in Nursing" brings into nursing a vital, evolving, and politically complex set of discussions that have informed other disciplines. She raises the question of who is speaking when texts in nursing refer to "nurses" or "we nurses." By posing the problem of which voices are actually heard in nursing, she also raises the more complex question of how the ways we organize our theoretical discourses both make possible and silence some perspectives—for example, those of nurses of color. Simultaneously, she poses the necessity of seeking coalitions while raising and honoring differences in political work that seeks structural transformation. These challenges are addressed in many of the other chapters, such as those by Gray, O'Neill, Allman, and Skillings.

How the complexities of voice and perspective, including commitments to specific views of social justice, do and can inform our research is the question taken up by Allen's chapter. He begins with the assertion that most feminist standpoints rule out the possibility of relativism by asserting the preferability of situated knowledges that are not sexist or racist. He then explores traditions in the philosophy of science that might prove helpful to nurses who are committed to the generation of scholarship grounded in perspectives that take explicit positions on gender, race, and class oppression. These themes have been raised frequently within the three conferences on feminist and critical perspectives in nursing and operate within many of the papers in this collection (from the second of the three conferences). Bunting and Henderson, for example, raise the problem of "alternative explanations" of experiences articulated by women; similarly, Condon, Hiraki, and others explore the implications of the language within which we form our descriptions, explanations, and goals of nursing. In listening to and reviewing these works, we have been fortunate. It is a gift to meet nurses who are committed to critical scholarship and practice. And the insights that are shared in this collection have pushed the boundaries of critique in nursing, challenging each of us to reexamine issues and silences in our own work. Here we are pushed to reexamine the politics of privilege in our own constructions, noticing, for example, how many of us are white, or middle class, or heterosexual. By learning to situate ourselves, to locate our voices in specific bodies that have been formed by specific sociocultural practices, we learn to see that our work is part of larger social constructions and that, through our work, we also act or have agency in the social world.

We hope that these papers function in multiple ways. Nurses who have contributed to this collection have "self-consciously situated themselves at vulnerable conjunctional nodes of ongoing disciplinary discourses where each of them posits nothing less than new objects of knowledge, new praxis of

. . . activity, new theoretical models that upset or at the very least radically alter the prevailing paradigmatic norms" (Said, 1986). This makes transitional work in nursing scholarship an important part of nursing praxis.

REFERENCES

Alexander, J. (1991). Sociological theory and the claim to reason: Why the end is not in sight. *Sociological Theory* 9(2), 147–153.

Flax, J. (1989). *Thinking fragments: Psychoanalysis, feminism, and postmodernism in the contemporary west.* Berkley: University of California Press.

hooks, b. (1991). *Yearning: Race, gender and cultural politics.* Boston: South End Press.

Said, E. (1986). Orientalism reconsidered. In F. Barker et al. (Eds.), *Literature, politics and theory* (pp. 210–229). New York: Methuen.

Tong, R. (1989). *Feminist thought: A comprehensive introduction.* Boulder: Westview Press.

Thompson, J. (1987). Critical scholarship: The critique of domination in nursing. *Advances in Nursing Science* 10(1), 27–38.

Janice L. Thompson

Feminism, Relativism, and the Philosophy of Science: An Overview

David G. Allen

INTRODUCTION

This chapter introduces some key issues in the feminist philosophy of science and attempts to increase our understanding of what a body of research based on feminist philosophy would look like.

Those of us committed to generating knowledge supportive of and consistent with emancipatory communities often find ourselves in a quandary: deeply skeptical of any claim to "authoritative" knowledge, we often lapse into various forms of relativism. Not wanting to claim too much for our research, we claim too little. While it is important not to overgeneralize the relevance of our work for fear of its colonialist potential, we tend to implicitly accept a view that marginalizes our work by leaving it either at a descriptive level or by believing its implications are limited to the context in which the study was actually conducted.

Relativism is not an option for feminists, however. Feminists and their supporters do not believe that feminism is just an *alternative* to racism, sexism, or classism (Harding, 1986; Fonow & Cook, 1991). It is *preferable*. But how does one argue that one's own science is preferable to another form of science without lapsing back into authoritarianism? Here, I will sketch out two themes that are keys to answering this question: first, what kind of scientific argument is necessary to simultaneously promote knowledge generation and protect against its oppressive potential (as well as to protect against its spread (Allen, Allman, & Powers, 1991)). A second, related theme has to do with the idea of "explanation." One reason so much feminist research has remained descriptive is the well-grounded fear of substituting the "researcher's" explanation for that of the persons being researched. Women and people of color have a long, terrible history of having their explanations supplanted by those of white, male scientists. A 1990 study by Rushton that asserted African Americans are more susceptible to AIDS because of a genetic predisposition to impulsive and aggressive behavior is only the most recent in a long line of such racist scientific enterprises (Rushton, 1989; Leslie, 1989). An equally long history of medical science providing biological explanations for women's inferiority has its current permutations in left-right brain attributions (Bleier, 1986).

The various feminist critiques of science have at their core a rejection of perceived relationships between patriarchy and science (Harding, 1986; Keller, 1985). There has also been increased concern with the interaction of dominant models of science and racist and class-based oppression (Fonow & Cook, 1991). Because current critiques have demonstrated how supposedly neutral or universalizing claims are shaped by the social position of scientists (among other aspects), these former "truths" have been "relativised."

These critiques have raised the question of what models of science can be created or adopted to avoid oppressive relationships. But as Harding and others have noted, the critique of the theory and practices of science from feminist and critical perspectives is far more developed than any elaboration of an alternative view of science. That we are clearer about what not to do than how we should proceed shouldn't be surprising or alarming. Contemporary philosophy of science emphasizes the social conditions within which scientific practices arise (Bernstein, 1983; Rorty, 1979; Benhabib, 1986). Unfortunately, few communities that have internalized the values and visions of feminism and critical theory have also generated much science. We will not know what a fully emancipatory science looks like until we have a fully emancipatory community.

This is not to suggest that we should abandon our efforts to criticize and reform science to concentrate primarily on issues of broader social justice. For one thing, the role of science in sustaining social injustices is too significant to ignore. In all likelihood, the same people who are articulating the critique of science are also addressing, in their own situations, other institutionalized practices of injustice.

What I will explore here, then, are two key issues in identifying a "preferable" science. First, there is the question of evidence or grounds or reasons: given that we have two competing theories or truth claims, what *kind* of evidence or reasoning should we use. The supposedly neutral contents of observation are no longer unproblematic (although we certainly don't want to abandon observational data). I will argue that we cannot rely upon any single or unique set of criteria or kinds of evidence—including the beliefs of oppressed people. Instead, we can only secure our arguments by understanding the social conditions in which they are debated. In this regard, the critical and feminist perspectives on *process* and *communication* are central to the establishment of an emancipatory science (Fay, 1987; Benhabib, 1987; Fraser, 1989; Lather, 1991).

Second, there is the problem of explanation: what is involved in explaining how or why something occurred. The current emergence of interpretive traditions, especially the more phenomenological perspectives such as grounded theory, in my view, simply beg this question. On what grounds do we prefer the interpretations and explanations of one group versus those of another? Under what conditions do we trust more the *explanatory* accounts of the mentally ill individual to those of the neurobehaviorist? The shaman to the oncologist? The woman to the psychiatrist? The political commitment of feminism and the belief in its preferability as a perspective do not allow us to escape these choices. However, in addressing *explanation*, I hope merely to highlight some of the issues underlying these alternatives just mentioned and how they might influence the construction of research programs.

The importance of the issues of evidence and explanation for feminist politics can be highlighted through a brief discussion of the problem of ideology. Other terms used to refer to this same notion are: *false consciousness, internalized sexism, self-defeating discourse,* or *denial* (Althusser, 1971; Sumner, 1979; Coward, 1985; Lichtman, 1982; Benhabib & Cornell, 1987). These are all current formulations concerning why "native" accounts are not necessarily preferable. Ideologies, we must remember, are not just sets of alternative belief systems. Some belief systems (e.g., those that value women or people of color as fully human) are, from our perspective, preferable to those that do not. The history of the term *ideology* (and its successors) embodies a notion of critique: ideologies (e.g., sociobiological notions of sexism or racism) are systematic misrepresentations or distortions (Thompson, 1984). They may be and often are fully and heartily believed and endorsed by their adherents, who need not be supposed to be acting on any conscious (or even unconscious?) bad faith. One can sincerely believe in racism even if that belief is not warranted. One can sincerely believe one is cured or is recovering, even when one is facing imminent death. One can honestly believe, as a woman, that one is genetically inferior and ought not embrace the rigors and stresses of public life.

Yet the phenomenological traditions and their adherents—as they emerge in nursing—limit us to simply describing belief systems (Lennon, 1990). The most sophisticated adherents, for example, can identify contradictions between beliefs or beliefs and actions, but, at the same time, they are relatively mute on the question of preferability or of systematic delusion. Thus, for both scientific and political reasons, we need a view of the explanation of racism and sexism that prefers Reverend Martin Luther King to Judge Clarence Thomas, Audre Lorde to Margaret Thatcher.

PROCESS CRITERIA FOR ESTABLISHING PREFERABILITY

The history of science should not be abstracted from the history of political emancipation (Harding, 1986; Forester, 1985; Foucault, 1979, 1980). The rise of modern science was part of a complex reaction to state imperialism and religious authoritarianism. The Protestant reformation that stressed individuals could read holy texts and establish their own relationships with the divine, the emergence of a merchant class as a model of social mobility, and the development of science as a form of discourse that could be used and assented to by any human being were all emancipatory projects. Like most such projects, however, they were gradually transformed into ideological straitjackets for later generations. The shattering of centralized religious authority and the social disruption of industrialization led to a model of extreme individualism, an abstract, single person without history and community. Science developed its own priesthood to interpret the divine text of nature to the unenlightened.

Scientific discourse and activity is a subset of broader, cultural discourse. Most philosophers since Kuhn have admitted that there is an interaction between cultural discourse and scientific discourse (Bernstein, 1983; Rorty, 1979, 1989). Harding, for instance, identifies a salient feature here which characterizes much talk about science as ideological: science wants to submit every activity to causal analysis except its own! On the other hand, one can talk about the social basis for the emergence of varying forms of scientific discourse as well as the effects of those discourses on broader social practices.

The reason I introduce this perhaps obvious point is to raise the issue of rationality. Rationality, in its broadest sense, refers to arguments which are recognized as being something other than mere personal opinion or the employment of force. What characterizes this difference is, of course, the heart of the matter. One factor which distorts our understanding of the preferability of feminist science is the extent to which a certain form of scientific rationality has been accepted as rationality per se. Even the term *rationality* is suspect for a feminist audience because it has been equated with specific Europatriarchal models of discourse (Bowles & Klein, 1983; Nicholson, 1989; Sayers, 1987). Feminist critiques want to acknowledge the role of emotion, for example, in rationality. One reason that scientific rationality failed to dominate European cultures to the extent that it did American discourse concerns the irrationality of fascism, which was a product of the best science of its age. The sociobiologic arguments of Darwin and his cousin Galton led directly to the ideas of racial purification. Since we manage to fight most of our wars on other people's soil, we are experientially less familiar with the horrors of these forms of scientific rationality—although during the Persian gulf war, only extreme censorship prevented it from entering the consciousness of white America. Indians who had suffered genocide in America through the virtual extermination of tribal cultures or those who suffered the perfectly rational, if nightmarish, science of the Tuskegee experiments or those who suffered imprisonment without trial and forfeiture of property for suspected Japanese ancestry during World War II find it less strange and often share feminists' suspicion of scientific rationality.

I believe that Habermas's view of democratic communicative situations and the feminist views of process can be combined to offer a model of social conditions under which truly alternative models of science can emerge and thrive—at least in Western, industrialized societies (Habermas, 1984; Fraser, 1987, 1989; Benhabib, 1986; Fay, 1987; Alford, 1985; Balbus, 1984; Love, 1991; Spivak, 1985).

In this regard, there are two sorts of communicative situations I must address. First, there is the commonplace, in which a group/community gathers to discuss issues within the contexts of relatively stable and taken-for-granted normative backgrounds. Such communicative situations might be viewed as nonrevolutionary interactions in which the social, political, and normative relationships among participants are not of primary focus. Those involved share enough common ground, perspectives, and values that the conversation can concentrate on resolving the issue and can be primarily directed away from the participants and toward the topic at hand.

Under these, most common, situations, Habermas (1984) proposes that rationality is approached through pursuit of two ideal conditions: autonomy and responsibility. Rationality refers to the confidence one can have in the outcome of the conversation. Consequently, it is not an "all or nothing" quality. The ideal conditions of autonomy and responsibility are probably rarely if ever fully achieved. Instead, autonomy and responsibility are "regulative ideals" toward which we constantly strive. *Autonomy*, which refers to the ability and willingness to participate openly in the conversation, requires being sufficiently self-reflective to understand one's own values, interests, needs, and inhibitions and to take them into account when interacting. *Responsibility* refers to ensuring that all participants can function autonomously by attending to group dynamics, knowledge imbalances, power differences, and so forth. Feminists have elaborated on these notions to emphasize two aspects ignored or neglected by Habermas: the *relationships*, the connectedness among participants, and the role of *emotion and intuition* understood not as threats to, but as supportive of, group rationality (Gilligan, 1889; Chinn & Wheeler, 1985; French, 1986).

Thus, when modified through the feminist insights, Habermas's notions of autonomy and responsibility are clarified and augmented to reflect the social and relational basis of communication. Autonomy is best supported in contexts within which one feels valued and loved. Responsibility requires attending to affective dimensions of interactions and to the intuitively appreciated patterns of connection and strain.

The notions of consensus and coalition are also important here; responsibility and autonomy require the balancing of separateness, difference, and connection. The more problematic this balance, the more conversations will lean toward more radical versions in which horizons are being reforged across communicatively achieved, rather than normatively secured, values. That is, the more difference there is among the values and experiences of group members, the more they will have to focus their attention on achieving a mutual understanding of individual perspectives. Value clarification must precede value negotiation. The focus will have to be first on the participants' worldviews, then on the topic at hand.

The above, then, is analogous to the distinction between Kuhn's notions of "normal" and "revolutionary" science (Kuhn, 1970). In normal science, conversations occur within a context of shared and taken-for-granted assumptions that allow discourse to proceed with a minimal level of self-reflection on the rules of discourse themselves. In revolutionary periods, however, the rules of logic, evidence, and normative assumptions come into dispute.*

---

*One reason the abortion debate can't proceed, for example, is that the discussion remains on the metalevel; until some common horizon is achieved, no movement is possible other than through force.

Feminist empiricists can often overturn sexist and racist science within the rules of normal empirical discourse; biased sampling, unclear variables, and faulty logic were among the errors in sociobiological science as critiqued by Ruth Bleier (1986).

For those who reject the empiricist paradigm, an increasingly important theme concerns the idea of "situatedness" (Haraway, 1988; Hekman, 1990). Sometimes viewed as a form of relativism, situatedness might be better understood as one moment within the formation of discursive communities. Rather than assuming the voice of "neutral authority" that ignores the social position of the author, "situated discourse" locates the speaker, specifying the personal, social, and cultural perspective of the author. In the absence of interpersonal conversation, this process of situating oneself might be understood as the opening gambit in an interaction. Locating oneself permits other participants to appraise how much of a horizon of beliefs, values, and experiences they share with the author or speaker (Pratt, 1984). The more divergent the horizon of author and reader, the more "wary" the reader is of conclusions offered; were the context interpersonal, more time and energy would be required to focus on communicatively achieved norms. It is important to emphasize that, like autonomy and responsibility, the notion of "situating oneself" is an ideal. One can never stand apart from one's position in order to describe it: the description of one's location is itself the product of a situated consciousness. Thus, the dialogical interpretation of situatedness maintains a vital openness to challenging and revising descriptions of the social "location" of participants.

The emphasis on situatedness reflects a historical shift away from a homogeneous set of speakers (who assumed their audience was equally homogeneous and shared their horizons). This is a product of (1) the increasing diversity of speakers (e.g., we have a more varied set of authors); (2) the awareness that the authors are not nearly diverse enough and can't be taken as unproblematically "representative"; and (3) especially, that the results of their conversation (monologue?) are often "applied" to individuals who were not involved in the original conversation at all.

For example, throughout the 1950s and 1960s, one could reasonably assume that the authors of scientific medical arguments were white, European males from fairly privileged social class positions. The "results" of their science were argued and assessed within a context of similar perspectives but often "applied" to groups (e.g., women or people of color) who were quite different and were not at all involved in the discussions of the merit of the work (Leavitt, 1984; Navarro, 1976; Waitzkin, 1983). Currently, diversification of scientific persons to include increasing numbers of women and people of color has shifted the conversation to the meta- or revolutionary level discussed above, in which the rules of discourse, of who gets to speak and under what conditions, are an important focus. Thus, academic discourse on feminist critiques of science arose. Similarly, these and others who had previously experienced the effects of having science applied to them, without full participation in its formation and review, increasingly questioned the "universality" of its premises and conclusions.

From this perspective, situatedness is not an implicit claim to relativity (i.e., that my work would be duplicated by and could only apply to persons exactly like me and the individuals I studied). Rather, it is part of a conversation that would include an *appraisal* of both the degree to which author, readers, and consumers shared a horizon and of whether any lack of overlap would influence its acceptability.* In other words, situatedness is an empirical and dialogical *question*, not a conclusion. It needs to be assessed, weighed, and discussed.

The more divergent the speakers (author, reader, or consumer), the more radical the nature of the communicative situation. As Benhabib points out these radical "discourses arise when the intersubjectivity of ethical life is *endangered*; but the very project of discursive argumentation presupposes the ongoing validity of a *reconciled* intersubjectivity" (in Rasmussen, 1990). In other words, the ideal communicative situation posited by Habermas and augmented by feminism assumes a commitment to securing intersubjective agreement through autonomy and responsibility. But in conditions of extreme difference or distrust, the premises for such discourse may not exist. This is precisely the situation in the Middle East peace conferences between Israeli and Palestinian groups; the current goal is to establish the ability and willingness to talk. This may be a precondition or a consequence of discussions of any particular topic, such as water rights or territorial control.

How do these themes address the problem of relativism? Science is inextricably linked to communities. Research must be viewed as an *argument*, as part of a dialogue within the community. Since the communities are often geographically dispersed, communication most often is through written and not interpersonal discourse. But within most Western contexts, rationality can only be assessed within the context of the communicative situation within which the dispute arose. Thus, we need to attend to the political institutions which support the community of scientists to maximize the ability for all citizens to participate therein and, by their participation, to pursue the ideals

---

*For example, if the author had been raised as a Methodist and the reader a Presbyterian, their horizons might diverge but not sufficiently to raise questions of mutual understanding of research on behavior interventions with Alzheimer's victims. If the research were on the role of religious beliefs in civil life, however, questions of mutual understanding might be raised.

of autonomy and responsibility (Lather, 1991; Lash, 1990). One moment in this process is the requirement to "situate" oneself, that is, to understand the position from which one speaks and to communicate that to one's audience. This permits an audience to appraise the extent to which they might expect to share a general perspective or alerts them to sources of possible divergence.

The call for critically informed action research by Thompson (1991), Lather (1991), and others is part of this same emphasis. If research, both as process and as reported, is conceived as an argument or dialogue, then it is critical that the participants include the people being researched. This involves more than simply calling them participants or coinvestigators; insofar as possible, they should be integrated into the conceptualization, design, execution, analysis, and reporting. Nor does this imply that results need be based upon a consensus or that the subjects' accounts are uncritically privileged, but that the process and reporting of the research reflect the different voices within the project.

Consequently, faced with competing claims, the most trustworthy are those which emerge from contexts which most closely resemble those described above. Of course, such conditions are precisely those envisioned by feminists as keys to a more just Western world.

Yet, even within the communicative situation as described above, how does one decide which explanations of human activity are preferable to others?

EXPLANATION

While it is both safe and laudatory to document women's voices through various forms of phenomenological and hermeneutic inquiry (Levesque-Lopman, 1988; Deegan & Hill, 1987), it is scientifically and politically more problematic to study *why* women say what they do. Immediately, certain specters rise from the mist: biological reductionism in which women are reduced to their reproductive organs; the nature/nurture controversy; and professional and patriarchal elitism that all too readily substitutes its understanding for women's own (Martin, 1987; Suleiman, 1986). Explanatory studies are necessary, however, to understand how to restructure social institutions so as not to reinforce or merely reframe current injustices (Thompson, 1984; Giddens, 1987; Bernstein, 1983).

Particularly apt is Anthony Giddens's theory of structuration—a theory I have used to explore the question of explanation individually and with students. Giddens (1987) offers a theory of what a comprehensive explanation would have to include. Because the theory provides a perspective on the relationship between individual action and social structures, it is especially helpful in determining the character of a comprehensive explanation. In addition, Giddens's theory permits an integration of biological information into the explanatory process, an integration which many social theories avoid or simply refuse to consider.

Further, Giddens has the advantage of familiarity with both European and British-American philosophies of science. Consequently, he endeavors to integrate disparate traditions such as Heideggerian hermeneutics, critical theory, and realist models of explanation. Since a full explanation of Giddens's model and current criticisms of it are beyond the scope of this chapter, I will highlight some of its theoretical features I have found most helpful.

Three Components of Giddens's Model

Giddens argues that a comprehensive explanation must include three dimensions: action (what the people being studied believe they are doing and why they are doing it), unintended consequences of action (consequences that "escaped" the knowledge or goals of the people [agents]), and unacknowledged conditions (resources that made the action possible but were not acknowledged in the actors' accounts). A terminological note is in order— I am using *people*, *agents*, and *actors* as synonymous terms that presuppose linguistically competent human beings.

Action. Explanation must *begin* with an account of what the actors are doing from their own perspective (Winch, 1958; Hookway & Pettit, 1978; Little, 1991; Lennon, 1990). This involves both description and explanation. For example, describing action differentiates between walking to work, sightseeing, or exercising to burn off calories or to reduce stress. Although the description often implies an explanation, this is not always the case. For example, the explanation of walking to work may be "because it's Monday and I'm due there by 8:00 A.M." or "I'm trying to reduce pollution and save money." Research strategies can include grounded theory or hermeneutic approaches (Roth, 1987; Madison, 1988).

Beginning with action from the actors' perspective is an asset from a critical perspective. First, it grants intelligence and agency to the people being studied; second, it makes more difficult an uncritical substitution or imposition of the researcher's explanation (Lather, 1991); third, it introduces the level of everyday activity that often provides the mediating process between "macro" level explanations, such as gender, race, or class, and individual behavior without reducing people to passive "effects" of social structure.

The study of action may involve several components. *Rationalization of action* refers to the agents' abilities to provide a "rationale' or a discursive account of what they are doing and why. *Reflexivity and monitoring of action* refers to the moment-to-moment, often subconscious, adjustment of individual behavior required to achieve a goal; for example, the motor reflexes and environmental scanning involved in walking down a sidewalk or in driving a car. Similarly, there are those adjustments that cannot be reduced to a set of discrete decisions and actions; for example, the internalized, field-dependent judgments studied by Pat Benner (Benner & Wrubel, 1989; Benner, 1985) and others. *Motivation of action* refers to the fact that action is goal directed; one is trying to keep a job and save money, lose weight, or avoid health problems. Motivation, however, need not be conscious; being socially acceptable, avoiding unpleasant feelings, and pleasing an internalized parent are all goals that may shape our behavior whether or not we recognize them consciously.

Unintentional Consequences of Action. Action, by definition, is intentional; almost all human behavior of interest (with the limited exception of purely reflexive feedback systems) is guided by goals or purposes. However, limited understanding, knowledge, and reflection result in our actions having consequences beyond our awareness or intention. I flip on a light switch intentionally to illuminate a room. My flipping on a light switch may also scare off a potential burglar or overload an electrical system and cause power outages. In another sense, I may be intending to hire only the "best qualified" candidate for a job but unintentionally discriminate against people of color or women. In response to such situations, our legal system makes radical distinctions between intentionality and unintentionality; for example, intentionally or unintentionally causing injury or death to others. The writing of history also comes to mind here. While history used to be written as the intentional outcomes of great men or, in the case of nursing history, of great women, increasingly it is being viewed as the unintentional consequences of much smaller and less global actions.

The notion of unintentional consequences helps account for certain forms of oppression without having to postulate or rely on more problematic "conspiracy theories." For example, a researcher or reader needn't assume that the writers of children's books were participating in a conspiracy to limit the social potential of women by reproducing stereotypes, that is, women characters caught up in stereotypically disempowered relationships with men or other conditions. Although some writers of children's books might have been so caught up, most of those writers probably never envisioned sexism as a consequence of their art.

Unacknowledged Conditions of Action. Unacknowledged conditions are resources that make the action being studied possible, but which are not recognized within the accounts of actors. Language and the material resources of privilege are apt examples here (McIntosh, 1988).

When one asks women about their experiences of menopause and how it shapes their daily actions, the responses received depend vitally upon the women's vocabulary (Dickson, 1990). Do the women asked have access to historical "folk wisdom" passed down by women generation after generation? How much do the women understand of the biology of menopause? How much of their view of menopause is shaped by the influence of biomedical perspectives reproduced in women's magazines? Language is a critical resource—it is central to both self-concept and the possibility of change. The U.S. government's "termination" programs that attempted to eradicate the languages and religious practices of Native Americans, for example, were based on the realization that control of language leads to control of populations (Swinomish Tribe, 1991). Whether meanings are expressed in verbal or nonverbal forms, they are incorporated into our understandings of ourselves and our visions of how the world might be. Consequently, regardless of whether or not the authors of children's books, the authors of college textbooks, or the writers of beer advertisements are *intentionally* sexist, their work must be challenged lest it influence the pool of meanings available for us and future generations. In this sense, much of the historical and mythological research of feminists has been directed toward recovering or creating more diverse and powerful vocabularies for women.

Tom Harkin, former 1992 presidential candidate, captured the material resources of privilege when he quipped that the problem with George Bush is that he was born on third base and thinks he hit a triple. Similarly, the racist and sexist political programs that promise, like the Colorado Ku Klux Klan leader, or Duke, Buchanan, or Bush, "equality for everyone, special consideration for none" are racist and sexist precisely because they fail to acknowledge the resources that *already* give men and whites unearned privileges (McIntosh, 1988). Their forefathers having slaughtered American Indians to gain the very land they stand on as they speak, these politicians speak out against "unfair" access of tribes to fishing and hunting resources. Having enslaved African Americans, passed generations of Jim Crow laws, segregated and underfunded school systems, they now decry the unfair advantages conferred by affirmative action. Having the privilege of seeing white male faces reflected at them in all media representations of success and power and, indeed, within the corridors of power themselves, they undermine the Equal Rights Amendment as unnecessary.

Another resource we rarely acknowledge due to the privilege of good health is physiological intactness. Our linguistic and physical competence is based upon adequate physical health.

As a category, the importance of unacknowledged conditions resides in its focus on the interaction between socially structured resources and individual human actions. We are not limited to just the accounts given by agents of what makes their actions possible. The symbolic and material resources of culture are critical to understanding human action and envisoning new social arrangements. Feminists have long understood this, of course, as exemplified in their efforts toward comparable worth, child care, and nonsexist media. Giddens's model simply helps us formulate and incorporate such conditions into our research programs.

CONCLUSION

As researchers, before we throw up our hands in despair, I must emphasize again that the themes discussed in this chapter should be seen as regulative ideals, as models to strive for. Giddens's model, for example, will rarely be fully incorporated into a single study; it is more helpful to think of applying it to *programs* of research. Similarly, we all conduct research under conditions usually not of our choosing, including constraints of tenure, funding sources, time, university bureaucracies, and so forth. Recall that I said we would fully understand the nature of emancipatory research only within the context of emancipatory communities. While I love my job, I am sad to report that I can't consider major research universities to be fully emancipatory either!

What the models of process and explanation provide, then, is an emerging vision of how to produce research that is resistant to the authoritarianism and imperialism of current research approaches. As we pursue these visions, we will no doubt find new ways in which our research efforts can serve oppressive purposes or discover old oppressive purposes reappearing in new forms. The only assurance available to us is commitment to participative, communicative ideals and the processes which can create and nurture them.

DISCUSSION QUESTIONS

1. Allen states that feminism cannot be relativistic because it is explicitly or implicitly presented as a *preferable* perspective. It is viewed as a "better" perspective than, say, racist or sexist approaches to research, theory, or practice. Summarize in your own words how the concept of "situatedness" can be used to balance the risks of relativism and authoritarianism.

2. Many feminist and phenomenological traditions emphasize the importance of women's understanding of their own lives. Research from these perspectives often elucidates women's view of, say, menopause or parenting. What are the strengths and limitations of approaches which limit themselves to explicating women's understanding of their own lives?

3. In nursing, as a health occupation, the realm of the "biological" is often regarded as more real, less socially implicated than psychosocial or cultural realms. Apply the model of explanation based on Giddens from Allen's chapter to both Allman's chapter, "Race, Racism, and Health," and Henderson's chapter on sociopsychoanalytic theory and women's health to develop your own ideas about how biological ideas play a role in our research on women. You might consider developing a rationale for a research proposal on an aspect of women's health that explores the relationships between the social functions of biological discourse and a feminist perspective on social-political context.

REFERENCES

Alford, C. F. (1985). Is Jurgen Habermas's reconstructive science really science? *Theory and Society, 14,* 321–340.

Allen, D. (1986). The use of philosophical and historical methodologies to understand the concept of "health." In P. Chinn (Ed.), *Nursing research methodology*, (pp. 157–168). Rockville, MD: Aspen.

Allen, D. (1987). Health, objectification and alienation: Critical social theory and the process of defining and attaining health. In M. Duffy & N. Pender (Eds.), *Conceptual issues in health promotion* (pp. 128–137). A report of proceedings of a Wingspread Conference. Indianapolis: Sigma Theta Tau International.

Allen, D. (1987). Critical social theory as a model for analyzing ethical issues in family and community health. *Family and Community Health 10*(1), 63–72.

Allen, D. (1989). Challenge: The influence of gender on nursing science. *Proceedings of the fifth nursing science colloquium: Strategies for theory development in nursing, V.* Boston University, 1988.

Allen, D. (1991). Applying critical social theory to nursing education. In N. Greenleaf (Ed.), *Curriculum revolution: Redefining the student-teacher relationship.* New York: National League for Nursing.

Allen, D., Allman, K. M., & Powers, P. (1991). Feminist nursing research without gender. *Advances in Nursing Science 13*(3), 49–58.

Allen, D., Diekelmann, N., & Benner, P. (1986). Three paradigms for nursing research: Methodological implications. In P. Chinn (Ed.), *Nursing research methodology* (pp. 23–38). Rockville, MD: Aspen.

Althusser, L. (1971). Ideology and ideological state apparatuses: Notes towards an investigation. In *Lenin and philosophy* (pp. 127–186). New York: Monthly Review Press.

Balbus, I. D. (1984). Habermas and feminism: (Male) communication and the evolution of (patriarchal) society. *New Political Science, 13,* 27–47.

Benner, P. (1985). Quality of life. *Advances in Nursing Science 8*(1), 1–14.

Benner, P., & Wrubel, J. (1989). *The primacy of caring.* Menlo Park: Addison-Wesley.

Benhabib, S. (1986). *Critique, norm, and utopia: A study in the foundations of critical theory.* New York: Columbia University Press.

Benhabib, S. (1987). The generalized and concrete other: The Kohlberg-Gilligan controversy and moral theory. In E. F. Kittay & D. Meyers (Eds.). *Women and moral theory,* (pp. 154–177). Totowa, NJ: Rowman & Littlefield.

Benhabib, S., & Cornell, D. (Eds.). (1987). *Feminism as critique.* Minneapolis: University of Minnesota Press.

Bernstein, R. (1983). *Beyond objectivism and relativism.* Philadelphia: University of Pennsylvania Press.

Bleier, R. (1986). *Science and gender: A critique of biology and its theories about women.* New York: Pergamon Press.

Bowles, G. (1984). The uses of hermeneutics for feminist scholarship. *Women's Studies International Forum, 7*(3), 185–188.

Bowles, G., & Klein, D. (Eds.). (1983). *Theories of women's studies.* London: Routledge, Kegan & Paul.

Campbell, J., & Bunting, S. (1991). Voices and paradigms: perspectives on critical and feminist theory in nursing. *Advances in Nuring Science 13*(3), 1–15.

Card, C. (1986). Oppression and resistance: Frye's politics of reality. *Hypatia*, *1*(1), 149–166.

Chinn, P. L., & Wheeler, C. E. (1985). Feminism and nursing: Can nursing afford to remain aloof from the women's movement? *Nursing Outlook*, *33*(2), 74–77.

Chodorow, N. J. (1985). Beyond drive theory: Object relations and the limits of radical individualism. *Theory and Society*, *14*(3), 271–319.

Collins, P. H. (1989). The social construction of black feminist thought. *Signs*, *14*(4), 745–773.

Coward, R. (1985). *Female desires: How they are sought, bought and packaged.* New York: Grove Press.

Deegan, M. J., & Hill, M. (Eds.). (1987). *Women and symbolic interaction.* Boston: Allen & Unwin.

Dickson, G. L. (1990). A feminist poststructural analysis of the knowledge of menopause. *Advances in Nuring Science 12*(3), 15–31.

Fay, B. (1987). *Critical social science: Liberation and its limits.* Ithaca, NY: Cornell University Press.

Fee, E. (1986). Critiques of modern science: The relationship of feminism to other radical epistemologies. In R. Bleier (Ed.), *Feminist approaches to science* (pp. 42–56). New York: Pergamon Press.

Fonow, M. M., & Cook, J. A. (1991). *Beyond methodology: Feminist scholarship as lived research.* Bloomington: Indiana University Press.

Forester, J. (Ed.). (1985). *Critical theory and public life.* Cambridge, MA: MIT Press.

Foucault, M. (1979). *Discipline and punish: The birth of the prison.* New York: Vintage.

Foucault, M. (1980). *The history of sexuality* (Vol. I). New York: Vintage.

Fraser, N. (1987). What's critical about critical theory? The case of Habermas and gender. In S. Benhabib & D. Cornell (Eds.), *Feminism as critique* (pp. 31–56). Minneapolis: University of Minnesota Press.

Fraser, N. (1989). *Unruly practices: Power, discourse and gender in contemporary social theory.* Minneapolis: University of Minnesota Press.

French, M. (1986). Beyond power: Women, men and morals. *The Women's Review of Books*, *IV*(1), 20–21.

Giddens, A. (1987). *Social theory and modern sociology.* Stanford, CA: Stanford University Press.

Gilligan, C. (1989). *Making connections: The relational worlds of adolescent girls at Emma Willard school.*

Habermas, J. (1984). *The theory of communicative action* (Vols. I & II). Boston: Beacon Press.

Haraway, D. (1988). Situated knowledges: The science question in feminism and the privilege of partial perspective. *Feminist Studies, 14*(3), 575–599.

Harding, S. (1982). Is gender a variable in conceptions of rationality? A survey of issues. *Dialectica 36,* (2–3), 43–63.

Harding, S. (1986). *The science question in feminism.* Ithaca, NY: Cornell University Press.

Harding, S. (1987). The curious coincidence of feminine and African moralities. In E. F. Kittay & D. Meyers (Eds.), *Women and moral theory* (pp. 296–316). Totowa, NJ: Rowman & Littlefield.

Harding, S. (1989). Taking responsibility for our own gender, race, class: Transforming science and the social studies of science. *Rethinking Marxism, 2*(3), 8–19.

Hekman, S. (1990). *Gender and knowledge: Elements of a postmodern feminism.* Boston: Northeastern University Press.

Held, D., & Thompson, J. (Eds.). (1989). *Social theory of modern societies: Anthony Giddens and his critics.* New York: Cambridge University Press.

Held, V. (1985). Feminism and epistemology: Recent work on the connection between gender and knowledge. *Philosophy & Public Affairs, 14*(3), 296.

hooks, b. (1984). *Feminist theory: From margin to center.* Boston: South End Press.

Hookway, C., & Pettit, P. (Eds.). (1978). *Action and interpretation.* New York: Cambridge University Press.

Jaggar, A., & Bordo, S. (Eds.). (1989). *Gender/body/knowledge: Feminist reconstructions of being and knowing.* New Brunswick, NJ: Rutgers University Press.

Keller, E. F. (1985). *Reflections on gender and science.* New Haven, CT: Yale University Press.

Kuhn, T. (1970). *The structure of scientific revolutions* (2nd ed. enl.). Chicago: University of Chicago Press.

Lash, S. (1990). *Sociology of postmodernism.* New York: Routledge.

Lather, P. (1991). *Getting smart: Feminist research and pedagogy with/in the postmodern.* New York: Routledge.

Leavitt, J. (Ed.). (1984). *Women and health in America.* Madison: University of Wisconsin Press.

Lennon, K. (1990). *Explaining human action.* LaSalle, IL: Open Court.

Leslie, C. (1989). Scientific racism: Reflections on peer review, science and ideology. *Social science and Medicine 31*(3), 891–912.

Levesque-Lopman, L. (1988). *Claiming reality: Phenomenology and women's experience*. Totowa, NJ: Rowman & Littlefield.

Lichtman, R. (1982). *The production of desire: The integration of psychoanalysis into marxist theory*. New York: Free Press.

Little, D. (1991). *Varieties of explanation*. San Francisco: Westview Press.

Lorde, A. (1984). The uses of anger: Women responding to racism. In *Sister outsider* (pp. 124–133). Trumansburg, NY: The Crossing Press.

Love, N. S. (1991). Ideal speech and feminist discourse: Habermas revisited. *Women & Politics, 11*(3), 101–122.

Madison, G. B. (1988). *The hermeneutics of postmodernity*. Bloomington: Indiana University Press.

Manicas, P., & Secord, P. (1983). Implications for psychology of the new philosophy of science. *American Psychologist*, 399–413.

Martin, E. (1987). *The woman in the body: A cultural analysis of reproduction*. Boston: Beacon Press.

McIntosh, P. (1988). White privilege and male privilege: A personal account of coming to see correspondences through work in women's studies. Working Paper No. 189 (pp. 1–15); Wellesley College.

Navarro, V. (1976). *Medicine under capitalism*. New York: Prodist.

Nicholson, C. (1989). Postmodernism, feminism, and education: The need for solidarity. *Educational Theory, 39*(3), 197–205.

Pratt, M. B. (1984). Identity: Skin, blood, heart. In E. Bulkin, M. B. Pratt, & B. Smith (Eds.), *Yours in struggle: Three feminist perspectives on anti-semitism and racism* (pp. 11–61). Brooklyn, NY: Long Haul Press.

Rasmussen, D. M. (1990). *Reading Habermas*. Cambridge, MA: Basil Blackwell.

Rorty, R. (1979). *Philosophy and the mirror of nature*. Princeton, NJ: Princeton University Press.

Rorty, R. (1989). *Contingency, irony and solidarity*. New York: Cambridge University Press.

Rose, H. (1989). Talking about science as a socialist-feminist. *Rethinking Marxism, 2*(3), 26–29.

Roth, P. (1987). *Meaning and method in the social sciences*. Ithaca, NY: Cornell University Press.

Rothenberg, P. (1990). The construction, deconstruction, and reconstruction of difference. *Hypatia, 5*(1), 42–57.

Rushton, P., & Bogaert, A. F. (1989). Population differences in susceptibility to AIDS: An evolutionary analysis. *Social Science & Medicine 28*(12), 1211–1220.

Sayers, J. (1987). Feminism and science—Reason and passion. *Women's Studies International Forum, 10*(2), 171–179.

Spivak, G. C. (1985). Feminism and Critical Theory. In P. Treichler, C. Kramarae, & B. Stafford (Eds.), *For alma mater: Theory and practice in feminist scholarship* (pp. 119–142). Chicago: University of Illinois Press.

Street, A. F. (1989). *Thinking, acting, reflecting: A critical ethnography of clinical nursing practices.* Unpublished manuscript.

Suleiman, S. (Ed.). (1986). *The female body in western culture.* Cambridge, MA: Harvard University Press.

Sumner, C. (1979). *Reading ideologies.* New York: Academic Press.

Swinomish Tribe. (1991). *A gathering of wisdoms.* La Connor, WA: Swinomish Tribal Community.

Thompson, J. (1981). *Critical hermeneutics: A study in the thought of Paul Ricoeur and Jurgen Habermas.* New York: Cambridge University Press.

Thompson, J. (1984). *Studies in the theory of ideology.* Berkeley: University of California Press.

Thompson, J. L. (1987). Critical scholarship: The critique of domination in nursing. *Advances in Nursing Science, 10*(1), 27–38.

Thompson, J. L. (1990). Hermeneutic inquiry. In L. Moody (Ed.), *Advancing nursing research through science* (Vol. II). Newbury Park, CA: Sage.

Thompson, J. L. (1991). Exploring gender and culture with Khmer refugee women: Reflections on participatory feminist research. *Advances in Nursing Science, 13*(3), 30–48.

Waitzkin, H. (1983). A marxist view of health and health care. In Mechanic, D., *Handbook of health, health care and the health professions* (pp. 503–528). New York: Free Press.

Wheeler, C., & Chinn, P. (1985). *Peace and power: A handbook of feminist process.* Buffalo, NY: Margaretdaughters, Inc.

Winch, P. (1958). *The idea of a social science and its relation to philosophy.* London: Routledge, Kegan Paul.

2

Identity Politics, Essentialism, and Constructions of "Home" in Nursing

Janice L. Thompson

I think of how I just want to feel at home, where people know me; instead I remember. . . that home was a place of forced subservience and I know that my wish is that of an adult wanting to stay a child; to be known by others, but to know nothing, to feel no responsibility (Pratt, 1984, p. 12).

INTRODUCTION

In this paper, I explore a series of conversations that have emerged in recent multidisciplinary literature. For me, these discussions raise issues and questions that are closely related to nursing's historical struggles for identity. However, I recognize that my choice of topic also reflects my personal struggles with identity. It is therefore necessary to situate myself in this text, so that readers can judge for themselves whether my experiences and my subjectivity as a nurse speaks to them.

I grew up in a white, middle-class home in the midwest of the United States. My father's background was mostly middle class, and my mother's background was working class and working poor. Christianity was an important influence in my home during my early childhood, but during later years my mother subtly helped me to explore new terrain. I later learned that she had always been a free thinker when we were young and that it had been difficult for her to express this iconoclasm within the confines of her Baptist family and my father's Baptist family.

When I was young, my mother hung a large prominent sign at our kitchen table: "Love one another." She taught us to respect other people. Although I grew up in a predominantly white suburban neighborhood, I remember my mother teaching me that we were never to use specific racist words and that we should not laugh when some members of our extended family made racist jokes. Her silence in these situations was deadly.

My father helped me to believe that I could do anything I wanted to do. He demonstrated this belief as a role model through his single-minded hard work. He became a successful businessman and absorbed the white establishment's construction of the patriarchal family and the gender politics that this implied. For the most part, I believe that he enjoyed and felt at home in the old boys' networks and in the halls of power. I have mixed memories of my father which include tenderness, authoritarian displays of power, and absence.

My parents separated and divorced after I left home, and I struggled to stay connected with each of them in new and different ways. Although many dynamics in my family were sexist and oppressive, others were loving, playful, and fun filled. I feel deeply connected to my family, to both of my parents, and to my brother and sister. I was also able to resolve some of the anger I felt toward my father before he died, although I still hold some conflict and grief.

When I attended college, it never occurred to me that my privilege, my holding of a white middle-class position and the opportunity it gave me to attend a university, had been derived from my family's privilege and that this privilege had been derived from the workers whom my father employed. It never occurred to me that I was privileged at all. I wanted to learn the knowledge and skill necessary to practice nursing, and I worked diligently to complete my bachelor's degree. All of my instructors and nearly all of the students were white and no one ever mentioned this. Many of the faculty spoke about the history of exploitation in nursing and argued that nurses would continue to be exploited unless nurses became politically active. We were taught that nursing should become unified as a profession and that this would require political work to develop alliances with nurses holding various credentials and degrees of expertise. No one ever spoke explicitly about class or racial struggles within nursing.

After I finished school, I practiced medical-surgical nursing in a hospital in a predominantly white community. I was married to a middle-class white man, gave birth to my first child, and continued to work in the hospital. After my second year of practice, I became increasingly discouraged and demoralized by the gender politics I experienced from male patients, hospital administrators, and physicians. I decided that I was experiencing "burn out" and that I needed to return to graduate school. A year later, my family and I moved so that I could begin this next phase of my career.

It was during this period of my life that I experienced "conscientization," a painful, powerful shift in my consciousness, in my conscience, and in my understanding of my own subjectivity. I continued to practice in a hospital setting during graduate school to support my family and my study. In this quintessentially privileged place, graduate school, I studied, for the first time in my life, with minority women in nursing who spoke about racism and fought against it. I experienced an African-American male professor in the classroom. I did ethnographic work with Southeast Asian refugees. I was befriended by a lesbian who helped me to understand the compulsory character of heterosexuality in our society. I came to see my own privilege against the backdrop of others whose exploitation made it possible for me to acquire "advanced knowledge and skills." I came to see my complicity in the structures of dominant culture, and it nearly destroyed my identity as a person and as a nurse. Pratt (1984) speaks about the danger of leaving students in this phase of conscientization.

> I did not feel that my new understanding simply moved me into a place where I joined others to struggle with them against common injustices. Because I was implicated in the doing of some of these injustices, and I held myself, and my people, responsible, what my expanded understanding meant was that I felt in a struggle with myself, against myself. This breaking through did not feel like liberation but like destruction (Pratt, 1984, pp. 35–36).

I am grateful that in my graduate work I was politicized by male and female professors who taught me to link both my privilege and my oppression as a nurse with structural features of society. These experiences taught me how to connect my own subjectivity with the structures and injustices of the social world so that I could struggle against those injustices rather than be paralyzed by them. In this context, I longed many times for the security and naiveté of my earlier years, when I just wanted to go "home." Gradually, I realized that home had been a construction developed for me in my first years as a student by experienced nurses. I saw that I could feel safe there because many other things had been suppressed or repressed.

Now I recognize that my years of graduate school were galvanizing years of struggle, when I was shown how to see aspects of my subjectivity that had been denied. I was taught then how to link my own conflicts with other related struggles and how to recognize my own participation in dominant culture. I see now that my life has been changed by these experiences and that my current concerns for identity politics in nursing are an extension of all these aspects of my past.

I situate myself in this work, then, by saying that I am white, I have been a registered nurse for 17 years, I am 40 years old, I have been married to the same man for 20 years, I have two children, and I teach in nursing and women's studies in a predominantly white public university in New England. Although I can recite these multiple aspects of my identity, I no longer believe that they add up to a completely coherent or unified self. I know that there are fragments of myself which operate in multiple and diverse ways, always in relation to others, sometimes consciously, sometimes unconsciously, to provide me with what I understand as my subjectivity. In the classroom, I work with students to explore the dynamics of colonization, sexism, racism, classism, and heterosexism in nursing and in our culture. I realize that while there is privilege in my life, I am trying to act and live with care, responsibility, and justice. I don't want to become paralyzed by the recognition that very few persons with my skin color and other sorts of privilege have ever avoided the pattern of becoming a colonizer.

IDENTITY POLITICS AND NURSING

Identity politics is one loosely defined school of thought which. . .attempt(s) to find for collective action a basis that doesn't marginalize lived experience, especially that of oppressed peoples, a basis which doesn't abstract away the complexity and contradictions embedded in human subjectivity (Bromley, 1989, p. 208).

The term *identity politics* gained currency in multidisciplinary literature during the mid 1980s and enjoys a mixed audience today. Among some cultural critics, identity politics is "uncool" (hooks, 1991, p. 20), and among others, it poses both important possibilities and significant limitations (Giroux, 1992). But the questions and issues raised in identity politics are part of the terrain that nursing and other communities of people are currently exploring (Phelan, 1989). Nurses can certainly learn important insights from these explorations.

Identity politics owes a great deal of its origin to feminist women of color, gays, and lesbians who have insisted on the celebration of multiple identities, noticing that each of our identities is constructed around the categories of race, gender, class, and sexual orientation. Identity politics connects the material conditions of people's lives to their individual subjectivity, linking the societal and the personal. Insights generated by identity politics include "the recognition of a self that is multiplicitous, not unitary; the recognition that differences are always relational rather than inherent; and the recognition that wholeness and commonality are acts of will and creativity, rather than passive discovery" (Harris, 1990, p. 581).

In identity politics, any attempt to create political alliances across differences is seen as a historical and social construction which posits common or collective concerns for people with multiple, crisscrossing identities. Identity politics has attempted to find ways to build these alliances without marginalizing differences and without glossing over the complexities of people's multiple identities.

During the mid 1980s, as many nurses began to question the scientific project of theorizing in nursing, identity politics may have influenced nursing itself. An earlier generation of white privileged nurses had theorized a way of constructing a collective paradigm for nursing. Beginning from their own experiences, these theorists abstracted about health, nursing, and people in context. This phase of theorizing was tied to a predominantly white, privileged professional agenda which sought to secure nursing's professional status through the development of scientific expertise. Nursing researchers were taught to develop and use theory as other privileged members of scientific communities had before. The creation and use of theory as a commodity and its circulation and consumption, particularly in predominantly white schools of nursing, then created a sense of shared, common reality for some nurses. The theories of/for nursing functioned then as constructions which provided a sense of "home" for some nurses.

In identity politics, this construction of "home" is noticed (de Lauretis, 1986). First, it is important to acknowledge that the desire for home is real and that a sense of shared community and belonging provides security. In identity politics, however, constructions of home are politicized by demonstrating both their enabling and repressive functions.

[Identity politics] claims that. . .a secure feeling of being at home is necessarily founded on repression: it depends on suppressing awareness of the differences among people, on refusing to see who is excluded from the home. However

expansive and inclusive a home may feel from within, membership is inevitably contingent on characteristics only a restricted set of people possess. The use of the term "repression" then refers here to both the barring of certain people and the stifling of one's own knowledge of them (Bromley, 1989, p. 209).

During the 1970s and the 1980s, nursing theory circulated representations of health, nursing, people, and context that functioned paradoxically. On the one hand, privileged nurses sought through these and other strategies to secure their own location within an industry increasingly dominated by medicine and corporate dynamics. On the other hand, these theories attempted to abstract away from the particular, to make universalizing claims that left behind specifics like gender, race, class, and sexual orientation. The circulation and consumption of nursing theories may have created a sense of shared community among some privileged nurses, who then were never predisposed to listen to minority voices or to notice the dynamics of repression within themselves or within the privileged representations of nursing.

Identity politics in nursing interrupts this situation. It notices what has been repressed, both within the individual and within the group claiming a unitary identity. Identity politics first acknowledges that identity is not static, but fluid and changing. This problematizes any attempt to construct identity through essentializing definitions of nursing or through taxonomies, universalizing theories, or essentialist claims regarding the "object" of nursing practice. Identity politics also maintains that identity is not unitary, but fractured and split by the different positions one occupies, by the different members of the group, by the parts of oneself that are repressed, or by the members of the group who are silenced.

Identity politics in nursing then may come to include those discourses which reclaim subjugated knowledges in nursing, discourses which return the lived experience of nurses to the center of nursing identity and discourses which don't abstract away the complexity and contradictions embedded in nurses' subjectivity. This *may* include current narratives about caring in nursing (Benner, 1991; Watson, 1990).

Nurses, however, do have a great deal to learn from other communities who have engaged in identity politics. In this regard, I am concerned by current attempts to revalorize subjugated knowledges in nursing, to revalorize care and clinical expertise without a concurrent effort to link these aspects of "our" subjectivity to structural features of society. I do not believe that nurses can establish collective identity or shared community unless privileged nurses become conscientized about their own privilege, inclusive of class, race, ethnicity, and sexual orientation as well as gender. "Identity politics differs from apolitical psychologizing of the social world in that analysis does not end with experience: it continues by contextualizing experience, *relating it to structural factors*" (Bromley, 1989, p. 209, italics added).

Identity politics in nursing may avoid a slide back into metaphorically static, essentialized constructions of "home" if we can notice who and what is repressed in our constructions. This move demands that we keep connecting our own experiences as nurses to the structural features of our society (e.g., class, race, gender, and sexual orientation). Other communities have learned these insights, and their experiences with identity politics can be helpful exemplars for nursing.

ESSENTIALISM AND IDENTITY POLITICS IN OTHER COMMUNITIES

I am concerned here to understand whether or not such a diverse community as nursing can sustain a collective identity, without basing our identity on repressive constructions of home. It seems to me that those working within the feminist movement, within African-American liberation movements, and within the gay community have recently registered common insights about identity politics. These experiences can teach us important lessons in nursing.

I begin here by exploring an insight derived from recent sympathetic criticisms of feminist theory. In careful examinations of gender and knowledge, Hekman (1990) and Spellman (1989) explore ways in which most feminist theory replicated some of the same Eurocentric (white, Western, heterosexual, privileged male) biases of dominant culture in the West. How is it, for example, that the feminist movement finally posited a knowing (female) subject, which it turns out was theorized to be nearly as universal (read white, Western, middle class) as the male subject (standpoint) masked in humanism?

Recent insights into the pitfalls of theorizing about woman-centered subjectivity have registered among some feminists with a growing dread and an ever widening awareness about the dilemmas that occur in any theoretical project. Elizabeth Gross (1990) discusses this dilemma as follows:

> *Any theory of femininity, any definition of woman in general, any description that abstracts from the particular, historical, cultural, ethnic and class positions of particular women verges perilously close to essentialism. . .essentialism [posits] the existence of fixed characteristics, given attributes, and ahistorical functions which limit the possibilities of change and thus of social reorganization. . . [but] if women cannot be characterized in any*

general way. . . then how can feminism be taken seriously? What justifies the assumption that women are oppressed as a sex? If we are not justified in taking women as a category, then what political grounding does feminism have? (p. 341, 334).

While the feminist movement in the West began with a political agenda to end sexist oppression, it grounded this political agenda in essentializing, universalizing claims about the oppression of women. This political strategy quickly encountered challenges by women of color, working-class women, lesbians, older women, and physically challenged women who did not find their subjectivities reflected in the universalizing claims of the feminist movement.

The essentialism at work in particular constructions of feminism has been made clear by Audre Lorde, Angela Harris, bell hooks and others who have criticized white women for not only privileging patriarchy over issues of race, class, sexual preference, and other forms of oppression, but also for defining patriarchy and the construction of women's experiences in terms that excluded the particular narratives and stories of women of color. In this case, racial and class differences among women are ignored in favor of an essentializing notion of voice that romanticizes and valorizes the unitary experience of white middle-class women, who assumed the position of being able to speak for all women (Giroux, 1992, p. 208).

Identity politics within the feminist movement has moved rapidly away from essentializing constructions of home or discourses that make universal claims for all women without noticing difference, without linking differences to structural features of society. An earlier form of essentializing identity politics was unable to achieve community within the feminist movement. It seems unlikely that this model of constructing community will succeed in nursing.

Initially, identity politics offered a powerful challenge to the hegemonic notion that Eurocentric culture is superior to other cultures and traditions by offering political and cultural vocabularies to subordinate groups by which they could reconstruct their own histories and give voice to their individual and collective identities. . . . [But] forms of identity politics that forgo the potential for creating alliances among different subordinate groups run the risk of reproducing a series of hierarchies of identities and experiences which serve to privilege their own form of oppression and struggle. All too often this position results in totalizing narratives that fail to recognize the limits of their own discourse in explaining the complexity of social life and the power such a

*discourse wields in silencing those who are not considered part of the insider
group (Giroux, 1992, p. 298).*

These insights derived from the feminist movement have parallels in other
communities. Steven Seidman (1991) discusses related insights about essentialism and identity politics in the gay community. Recounting the history
of the 1980s and the institutional elaboration of the gay subculture, Seidman
presents a compelling discussion of his experiences as a gay activist. This
discussion parallels those found earlier in feminist literature and has important
implications for nursing.

Seidman (1991) notices that sometime prior to the 1980s, gay activists
began to deploy science to reverse the effects of regimes of power. As science
had created two master categories for the sexual self, heterosexual and ho-
mosexual, gay and lesbian activists began to use science to combat its own
stereotyped and stigmatized images. The experiences of gay and lesbian activists in this process are breathtakingly similar to those discussed by feminists.

> *The crystallization of an affirmative gay identity and community brought to
> the surface a new set of internal tensions and struggles. Legitimating ho-
> mosexuality, which meant building affirmative identities and communities
> around same-sex desire, did not necessarily entail challenging the core as-
> sumptions of the broader sexual order. Therefore, those desires and practices
> which were marginalized and censored within the dominant sexual regime for
> reasons unrelated to a homosexual choice of sexual object remained stig-
> matized. . . . Moreover, behind its universal claims to speak for all homo-
> sexually inclined persons were the values and social agenda of a narrow
> segment of this population. This agenda excluded or marginalized many who
> described themselves as lesbian or gay. The gay community thereby reproduced
> the forms of oppression that many of these marginalized groups—people of
> color, working-class people, those with disabilities—experienced in the broader
> social mainstream (pp. 182–183).*

For a time, it seemed important for the gay community to theorize gay
subjectivity, to tell a fairly Big Narrative, one capable of "valorizing" gay
identity. But eventually this move repeated the script of the dominant culture.
Seidman (1991) discusses more recent responses within gay/lesbian communities.

> *Insofar as the new affirmative gay construction projected being gay as the
> core, essential self-identity, it blinded gays to differences among them due
> (say) to race, class, gender, age, or ethnicity. These were often considered
> secondary characteristics yielding minor variations on the primary identity
> theme of being gay. I believed, as did other activists and intellectuals, that*

this view promoted an insular community and narrowly focused interest-group politics. This essentialist ethnic model of homosexuality may have been fruitful, even necessary in the 1970s for the purpose of community building and political mobilization. By the 1980s however—as the internal social differences exploded into gay public life and as the community came under attack by antigay crusaders—the social and political agenda seemed to require a shift away from an essentialist/ethnic model with its narrow interest-group politics. We needed to break down some of the exclusiveness between minority, feminist, and gay communities. This was not simply a matter of building a rainbow coalition by encouraging gays to grasp that they shared common interests with, say, African-Americans or Latinos. . . . Rather they needed to see that they were simultaneously identified by their racial/ethnic, gender, and class status or affiliation and that gays, like African-Americans or women, were simultaneously implicated in heterogeneous sexual, gender, racial/ethnic, and class struggles. To make this social and political shift requires a shift towards a concept of the self as exhibiting multiple, crisscrossing identities, social roles and interests (p. 183).

I find the parallels between these discussions of identity politics and the challenges facing nursing to be remarkable. I notice a period of time (roughly the 1970s to the 1980s) when it became important to invert the subordinate member of a binary. Wherever the opposition was found, there were efforts to theorize the underside (e.g., black/white, gay/straight, women/men, care/cure). I locate white feminist women in nursing who have participated in this process. I notice the scientistic development of nursing theory as an attempt to build community in nursing. I notice different attempts to build community in nursing in more recent white feminist nursing literature about a relational ethic of care. I recognize similar efforts to establish community in white feminist approaches that revalorize practical knowledge in nursing. Essentializing approaches to nursing identity have been an important moment in our lifetime. We are positioned in terms of these discourses; we were/are formed by these discursive practices. And how do we deal with the entanglement that presents itself when these essentialist interest-group forms of identity begin to explode?

Seidman (1991) offers some thoughts that seem relevant.

I don't think it was merely coincidental that the early 1980s simultaneously saw the rise of coalition politics in the gay community and the rise of social constructionism. Framing gay identity as an emerging sociohistorical event, as an unstable, contestable institutional/discursive production and strategy, provided gays with a rationale to begin to see themselves as having multiple identities, recognizing multiple, sometimes contradictory positions of social

power and oppression and seeing their own fight for sexual/social empow-
erment as connected to struggles around gender, race, ethnicity, class and
so on (p. 181, 183).

Within the feminist movement and the gay movement, identity politics have been "tricky." Much depends on the theories or the stories that are told. It matters, in other words, that the theories or narratives revalorize the subordinated member of a hierarchy, that they provide a political axiology for marginalized groups within dominant culture. However, it also matters that the stories are understood as social, historical constructions, practices of empowerment, attempts to develop collective identity and politics, "narratives with a moral intent"—and that these narratives help people to see their own struggles for empowerment *as connected to other related struggles.*

It seems to me that essentialist approaches to empowerment in nursing will simply be dismissed by those who do not find their subjectivities reflected in these constructions. Like other communities who have tried these strategies, we may discover that the revalorization of subjugated knowledges simply slides into another recursive replication of dominant culture. We may be able to avoid this slide if we engage instead in identity politics and if we learn to use political discourse to help us see that our subjectivities are simultaneously linked to class, race, gender, and other struggles.

CRITICAL PEDAGOGY AND NURSING EDUCATION

These lessons from identity politics raise significant questions for nursing education. While the development of identity in nursing remains an important function of nursing education, there is a need for a radically revised version of identity politics in nursing, "where identity politics based on essentialism is critiqued, while the connection between identity and politics is affirmed" (hooks, 1991, p. 20).

Critical educators have struggled with these questions and have explored strategies for helping students to develop identities that are fluid, politicized, and tuned into transformation. Giroux (1992), borrowing I believe from Anzaldua (1987), replaces the metaphor of "home" with the image of "borderlands" in his practice as an educator. Critical educators argue that if we wish to do something other than replicate the white establishment in nursing education, students will need to experience "borderlands" through the narratives of different people in our culture. These insights have been helpful to me as I meet students in the classroom and in the community.

Border pedagogy suggests not simply opening diverse cultural histories and spaces to students, it also means understanding how fragile identity is as it moves into borderlands crisscrossed with a variety of languages, experiences, and voices. There are no unified subjects here, only students whose voices and experiences intermingle with the weight of particular histories that will not fit into the master narrative of a monolithic culture. Such borderlands should be seen as sites for both critical analysis and as a potential source of experimentation, creativity, and possibility (Giroux, 1992, p. 209).

For others, identity politics requires the use of more than one metaphor. Bernice Reagon (1991) uses both the metaphors of "home" and of "excursions into borderlands" in coalition work.

Coalition work is not work done in your home. Coalition work has to be done in the streets. And it is some of the most dangerous work you can do. And you shouldn't look for comfort. Some people will come to a coalition and they rate the success of the coalition on whether or not they feel good when they get there. They're not looking for a coalition; they're looking for a home! They're looking for a bottle with some milk in it and a nipple, which does not happen in a coalition. You don't get a lot of food in a coalition. You don't get fed a lot in a coalition. In a coalition you have to give, and it is different from your home. You can't stay there all the time. You go to the coalition for a few hours and then you go back and take your bottle wherever it is and then you go back and coalesce some more. It is very important not to confuse them—home and coalition (p. 310).

In my work with students, I understand the need for constructions of "home." Some educators may argue that undergraduate students or novices can feel isolated and fragile until they are competent in the practice of nursing. These educators may say that undergraduate education or other primary socializations into nursing should provide a sense of security, shared identity, or "home."

But I do not wish to romanticize nursing education by equating it with repressive constructions of "home." Instead, I believe that nursing education works best when it helps students to move between "home" and "borderlands," where "home" includes all aspects of students' subjectivity that are known and familiar and "borderlands" includes all those stories about differences that have been repressed.

The very meaning of "home" changes with the experience of decolonization, of radicalization. At times home is nowhere. At times one knows only extreme estrangement and alienation. Then home is no longer just one place. It is locations. Home is that place which enables and promotes varied and ever-

changing perspectives, a place where one discovers new ways of seeing reality, frontiers of difference. One confronts and accepts dispersal and fragmentation as a part of the construction of a new world order that reveals more fully where we are, who we can become, an order that does not demand forgetting. Our struggle is also a struggle of memory against forgetting (hooks, 1991, p. 148).

There is a need for this kind of critical pedagogy in nursing education. Students are empowered when they develop identities that are tuned into transformation. Educators can assist in this process by helping students to see that their struggles for empowerment are connected to the struggles of other diverse people.

DISCUSSION QUESTIONS

1. This paper raises questions about the possibilities of sustaining common social and political agendas for nursing as an institution. What does Thompson mean by "essentialist" approaches to community and empowerment in nursing? What are some examples of essentialist strategies in nursing?

2. What does this paper suggest as an alternative way to build community in nursing? How does identity politics address differences based on race, class, gender, or sexual orientation? What would this mean for nursing and for patients?

3. Thompson argues that cultural politics in general now is focused on broad social transformations and that nursing is part of this process. Do you agree that identity politics as discussed here point toward the transformation of existing power structures (e.g. race, class, gender, and sexual orientation)? How should we as nurses participate in this process?

REFERENCES

Anzaldua, G. (1987). *Borderlands. La fronters: The new mestiza.* San Francisco: Spinsters/Aunt Lute.

Benner, P. (1991). The role of experience, narrative and community in skilled ethical comportment. *Advances in Nursing Science* 14(2), 1–21.

Bromley, H. (1989). Identity politics and critical pedagogy. *Educational Theory,* 39(3), 207–223.

de Lauretis, T. (1986). Feminist studies/critical studies: Issues, terms and contexts. In T. de Lauretis. (Ed.), *Feminist studies/critical studies.* Bloomington: Indiana University Press.

Giroux, H. (1992). Resisting differences: Cultural studies and the discourse of critical pedagogy. In Lawrence Grossbert et al. *Cultural Studies,* (Eds.), (pp. 199–212). New York: Routledge.

Gross, E. (1990). A note on essentialism and difference. In S. Gunew (Ed.), *Feminist knowledge as critique and construct.* London and New York: Routledge.

Harris, A. (1990). Race and essentialism in feminist legal theory. *Stanford Law Review,* 42.

Hekman, S. (1990). *Gender and knowledge: Elements of a postmodern feminism.* Boston: Northeastern University Press.

hooks, b. (1991). *Yearning: Race, gender and cultural politics.* Boston: South End Press.

Phelan, S. (1989). *Identity politics: Lesbian feminism and the limits of community.* Philadelphia: Temple University Press.

Pratt, M. B. (1984). Identity: Skin, blood, heart. In E. Bulkin, M. B. Pratt, & B. Smith (Eds.), *Yours in struggle: Three feminist perspectives on antisemitism and racism.* Brooklyn, NY: Long Haul Press.

Reagon, B. (1991). Coalition politics: Turning the century. In J. W. Cochran et al. (Eds.), *Changing our power: An introduction to women's studies.* Dubuque, IA: Kendall-Hunt.

Seidman, S. (1991). Postmodern anxiety: The politics of epistemology. *Sociological Theory* 9(2), 180–190.

Spellman, E. (1989). *Inessential women: Problems of exclusion in feminist thought.* Boston: Beacon Press.

Watson, J. (1990). The moral failure of the patriarchy. *Nursing Outlook, 38,* 30–33.

3

Race, Racism, and Health: Examining the "Natural" Facts

Karen K. Maeda Allman

INTRODUCTION

The National Institutes of Health (NIH) (1990) has reflected current national concerns with race and race relations in its 1990 call for "added attention (where feasible and appropriate) to the inclusion of minorities in study populations for research" (p. 10). The NIH also mandated that any studies which lack representation of "minorities" and "women" give a rationale for this lack. I have sought within this paper to examine discourses on race and on race and health, asking not what race is nor what the true relationship between race and health is, but rather, these three questions: (1) What is the discourse on race? (2) What are possible subject locations within this discourse? (3) Where are the silences? I will conclude with a discussion of four important shortcomings in research on race and health.

The author would like to acknowledge the help and support of David Allen in preparing this chapter.

RACE AND DISCOURSE

Recently, I began an examination of what has been said about race and health in the scientific medical and nursing literatures. My previous educational experiences had contained very little about race, culture, and health beyond the level of a few interesting anecdotes, for example, about infant care beliefs of Mexican Americans or the occasional frightening statistic about the higher infant mortality rate among African Americans. The work of medical anthropologists such as Noel Chrisman, psychiatrists with medical anthropology training and interests such as Arthur Kleinman, and nurse anthropologists such as Madeline Leininger was, of course, available for those interested in "culture," but at that time very little of it had trickled into my own educational settings. My ongoing critical examination of the last ten years of nursing periodicals and texts indicates that this is in a large part true of nursing education and research in general.

As a graduate student, I was steered away from studying nonwhite persons,* as these kinds of studies were, it was explained to me, complicated by those populations' cultures. This was especially true if we did not have "normative" data on a particular subject first, before we thought about working with the confounders or barriers of culture. Once the norm was established, using as homogeneous a group as possible, "other" groups, by definition too different to be included in the norm, could then be compared to this standard. (The paradigm case for this is IQ testing, often discussed in the context of cultural difference and occasionally used to demonstrate a heirarchy of racial development.)

I was not surprised to find that comparatively little else seemed to have been written on the health of nonwhite persons. What is interesting to me now is that, at the time, I did not find this fact particularly remarkable, even though I myself am not a white person.

The National Institutes of Health mandate, taken alone, can similarly be read to imply a previous silence about race in health research. Certainly, such silences exist, and part of my task is to identify where these silences exist and how they might function. I was quite interested to find that, in

---

*White, rather than "Caucasian" or "European American" or other term, will be used to delineate a type of social and political space and to attempt to provide some distance from naturalized physiological and ethnicity based connotations of other words. Further, "Caucasian" may also include people otherwise designated as Ainu, East Indian, and Hispanic or Latino, to name only a few. How individuals choose to name themselves, however, should be their own prerogative.

fact, the silences have not been complete. Some readers at this point may be wondering why I have not undertaken the project of defining the "true" relationship of race and health. Isn't it critical to study whether race and health are related? Adding in the further variable of the provision of health-related services, we might also ask if health care is racist. Since inequities in health care access and in morbidity and mortality among races do exist, cannot we reduce these questions to those of impoverishment and forget the question of race altogether?

Consistently reducing the complex interrelationships among questions of race and health has lead us to inadequate solutions. Questions about the relationships between race and morbidity and mortality are old ones, which resurface from time to time in different guise. At the turn of the last century, the Irish were considered a "race," and considered racially more susceptible to rheumatic fever. This susceptibility was proposed to be linked genetically to red hair (Cooper & David, 1986). The gene, of which red hair was the distinguishing racial mark, was believed so significant that other influences, such as environmental factors, were overwhelmed by it. That Irish immigrants to the United States did indeed have a higher incidence of rheumatic fever was proposed both as proof that the Irish were a race and as evidence that the Irish were "naturally" inferior. Today, Irish Americans are usually considered, at least by North Americans, as an ethnic or cultural group, not a race, and theories on genetic links between red hair and rheumatic fever are long out of favor. The discourse on race and health and their relationship has shifted from the Irish to a new subject.

Discourses can be thought of as multiple, discontinuous conversations, mediated by written, spoken, and enacted texts and separated by time and space (Foucault, 1977). This is not one story, but many. A discourse model (e.g., of science or theory) is at odds with more traditional, teleological, "grand" or master narratives of the progress of science, including the science of race. Foucault (1977) would label these, somewhat ironically, as "true discourses." They are true in as much as a complex web of power relations, embodied practices, and resistances holds them in place. Thus, the analysis does not stop at disproving the "truth" of the discourse on red hair, Irishness, and rheumatic fever, but moves on to examine the context of the times, the carriers of the discourse, its antecedents, and linkages with the production of similar hypotheses in the present.

The approach I have taken in examining this literature can be described as postmodern, in that I have been concerned with discourse analysis and de/construction, rather than with stories of "origins" or of fixed relationships between race and health. I am using de/construction to mean the process of taking apart to examine chains of associations in history, literature, science, culture, and the like, rather than as a way to find some hidden, fixed, ultimate meaning or final answer to one question. Multiple questions, positions, and degrees of power are possible in these types of analysis.

Contained within this type of de/construction are also the seeds of new ways of seeing and of hope for improving upon past mistakes. I contend, following Haraway (1988), that there is the possibility of critical, contestable, historically contingent knowledges about a world that are both material and symbolic. Race and health are associated with and have material consequences for real bodies and real people, even as meanings and consequences of race and health vary. Science and other forms of discourse on race and health are simultaneously social and semiotic, or meaning-producing, processes in which we bring all of ourselves to engage with other meaning-making actors in a living world. This living world, of course, includes our material and semiotic selves, our bodies. It is important not to confuse or collapse any living worlds with our own discourses and historically contingent scientific knowledges about them.

WHAT ARE SOME DISCOURSES ON RACE?

Race, like the genes that allegedly determine it, is often represented as a part or a property of individual bodies. Race is regarded as self-evident, common sense. This is the approach that biomedical research commonly takes to race: that race is an unchanging, "natural" fact of the body.

According to Polednak (1989), "*Races* are not artificial assemblages of 'types' but natural units or populations that undergo evolutionary change." (p.3). Yet, on the same page Polednak admits that race is an "imprecise" concept. North American immigrant groups of European origin are further described as "ethnic groups" that are "culturally distinct" rather than naturally so. Although gene frequency differences are noted among these groups, these differences are not usually regarded as denoting different racial groups at this time in history. The language of genetic difference is often invoked in differentiating the races as well, however. How is it that certain genetic differences, such as skin pigmentation, are held as significant in determining race and other genetic differences are not?

Another important question is, how many races exist? Many typologies of race, proposing three, five, twenty races or more, have been suggested, but little agreement among even biological scientists as to what exactly constitutes a race has been reached (Cooper & David, 1986; Polednak, 1989), though Polednak presents several competing and thoroughly complex examples. Are the Jews a race? Can the Japanese or Asians be considered a race?

The so-called three major races of man, caucasoid, mongoloid, and negroid, are said to be differentiated by variation in the frequency of the appearance of genes that determine blood groups and specific proteins (Polednak, 1989). Yet genetic tests are obviously not how an individual's race is usually determined, and health research on race rarely links a specific blood group or protein to a particular health outcome. Such outcomes would be anticipated to be distributed, though unevenly, among races anyway, as these genetic differences are not endemic to a race but vary in frequency among the races.

The oft-cited example of the "biological reality" of the races is, of course, sickle cell trait, which is often associated with Africans and African Americans. Sickle cell trait and sickle cell anemia do affect some members of these populations, and yet, on closer examination, the distribution of this trait seems to be not in the imagined "negroid race" as a whole, but present particularly among West Africans and their descendants. Furthermore, while the age-adjusted death rate of U.S. African Americans is higher than for white persons in nearly every major cause of death, African Americans and white Americans die from the same types of illnesses. Hemoglobinopathies accounted for 0.3 percent of excess African-Americans versus white deaths, adjusted for age, in 1977 (Cooper & David, 1986). The stereotype of African Americans as carriers of hemoglobinopathies, and thus as less healthy, has justified racial discrimination in employment on grounds of "health." An analogous though fictitious scenario would involve not hiring white persons on the basis of higher skin cancer rates or preferentially hiring Asian persons because Asian persons have a much lower rate of cystic fibrosis. A final consequence is the misdiagnosis of hemoglobinopathies, including forms of sickle cell anemia, in populations not considered Black, such as certain Indian and Saudi Arabian groups (Polednak, 1989).

I am not stating that differences in population subgroups do not exist, nor that such differences do not deserve research attention; rather I suggest that we reexamine the attributions that we make about these differences, their sources, and their consequences. Sometimes the difference may be seen as the very source of the consequence, as if the difference is the critical variable, and not the social context in which it occurs. Sociocultural contexts are also involved not only in reinforcing the difference but in constructing it in the first place. If one racial group has a higher morbidity and mortality, how is it that the race and not the social conditions that structure the relative distribution of resources by race is considered most salient?

SCIENCE AND NATURE

Gordon (1988) has noted that biomedicine, or modern, Western scientific medicine, is heavily influenced by naturalism. Naturalism presupposes a nature separate from culture and human consciousness. Nature is considered neutral, atomistic, universal, independent of time and space, and autonomous of society. While society and culture might apply to groups, (natural, autonomous) individuals preexist both. Nature is thought to be orderly, lawful, and predictable, and our emotions and subjectivity can only impede our understanding of nature. Bodies, and the diseases which affect them, exist separately from mind and spirit, are material, and thus are natural. Bodies are treated as nature's representative in human form, and race, as a property of bodies, is assigned to the category of nature.

The many advantages of a naturalist approach to biomedicine and nursing are probably obvious. An oft-cited additional advantage of the "neutral" biological approaches is the lifting of blame for illness from the sufferer. The advent of scientific approaches moved disease causation and treatment out of moral domains and into nature, where a dispassionate science might efficiently treat and cure it. However, biomedical discourse sometimes contributes to redefining social and cultural problems as biological problems either waiting for a technological fix or confirming the "natural" inferiority of a particular group. The supposed inferiority of a natural group (a race or a sex) is transformed from a social or political question up for public debate into a technical problem for the experts, or biomedical scientists, to *solve*.

The earlier discussion of Irish people provides a historical example. The living conditions of these immigrants were ignored in the quest to find a "natural" solution for a supposedly innate problem, a question of race. This Irish "genetics" problem was replaced with similar propositions about African Americans and then about Latin American genetics as these groups moved into particular socioeconomic niches and developed similar propensities toward rheumatic fever (Cooper & David, 1986). In each of these cases, the cause of disease was attributed to some innate factor endemic to one's race. If the group were more susceptible to the disease, it stood to reason that group membership, the "natural" fact of race, produced the disease. The obvious cure remains in the hands of the experts looking ever deeper for the cause within the bodies of the sufferers and not in living and working conditions. Disease and difference, in this case racial difference, become symbolically linked within both the popular and the scientific imagination.

Race, therefore, has become a problem for the scientist. Race, under naturalism, has to do with the body, or the stuff of nature. Sometimes race is conflated with ethnic identity, a sense of peoplehood based on shared national origins (Chrisman, 1991), or with culture. Both, as stated earlier, are posed as oppositional or irrelevant to nature. Racism, described by Yamato (1990) as "systematic mistreatment of one group of people by another on the basis of racial heritage" (p. 22), is another problem related to race. Racism, associated as much with social, cultural, and political aspects as with human consciousness is, under naturalism, not a concern of the biomedical scientist. Race, ethnic identity, and racism are not unrelated. However, the conglomeration of these under the rubric of race efficiently removes the possibilities for debate and action from the public arena to the scientific. Race thus becomes transformed from a social, political, historical, and cultural matter to a problem of nature to be solved by scientists.

THINKING BEYOND BIOLOGY

Omi and Winant (1986) proposed the term "racial formation" to describe flexibility and change in race and racial meanings over time. Various co-existing paradigms, including the previously discussed biological, ethnicity, and class-based theories, have appeared at particular historical moments. While some are currently favored over others, none have completely disappeared. The racial formation approach emphasizes the multiple, changing, sometimes contradictory themes that influence American ideas about race.

The ethnicity paradigm emerged in the 1920s as a challenge to previously held biologistic theories of race, including the de facto superiority of the "white race." Rather than comparing dubious, supposedly biologically determined racial characteristics, proponents of ethnicity theory concentrated on culture, migration patterns, social group membership, and descent (Omi & Winant, 1986). Weaknesses of ethnicity theory include its inability to account for norms external to the group, particularly in discussions of the eventual assimilation, lack of desire to assimilate, or failure of ethnic groups to assimilate into the so-called "melting pot" of American society. While language, country of origin, generation of immigration, and cultural differences were and are important in theoretical discussions of ethnic groups popularly considered "white," the same dominant "white" culture apparently does not consider such differences important, especially in relation to Americans designated as "black" (Omi & Winant, 1986) or "Asians." Further conceptual collapse has occurred in health research, where choice or breakdown of ethnicity is often Caucasian, Asian, Native American, African

American, and Hispanic, roughly analogous to the white, yellow, red, black, and brown "'races" of earlier days.

Social class-based theories (Omi & Winant, 1986) have also been proposed in the attempt to explain both ethnicity and race. Impoverishment and economic disequilibrium are viewed as producing racial inequality, and as impoverishment decreases, race ceases to be significant. Market forces thus are thought to act upon individuals equally, producing the illusion of racial discrimination though the root cause is economic discrimination. Class-based theories of race cannot explain why it is that members of certain racial groups are consistently overrepresented in impoverished groups, however. Omi and Winant (1986) similarly remind us that the members of the African-American middle class are still "black," with significant familial, cultural, political, and economic ties to impoverished African Americans. Political action on the part of African Americans provided for enhanced educational and employment opportunities for African Americans and other persons of color. Jobs, housing, and schooling were not, under Jim Crow segregation laws, denied to poor people, but to black people. Opportunities for poverty thus are a result of one's race, and not the reverse.

Joseph Scott proposes that race can more adequately be described as a permanent political class, like gender, which social class can amplify but which cannot be removed through marriage, class mobility, or education. Scott's analysis reminds us that race, like gender, is more closely identified with and projected upon the physical features of bodies.

Class-based theories to explain racial discrimination in health care provision (Funkhouser & Moser, 1990) are similarly inadequate. The artificial separation of race and class, not to mention gender, obscures differential opportunity structures organized by race and amplified by class. Put more simply, while being poor can increase one's chances for poor health, being nonwhite and female can increase one's opportunities to be poor and remain poor.

United States hospitals designated "for white persons only" under segregation did not treat any African-American persons, male or female, poor or not. Limited, poor-quality, or alienating educational and job opportunities maintain the overrepresentation of people of color within the economically disadvantaged and perpetuate limited access to health care. The nursing profession has itself practiced racial segregation not only within many of its schools, but also with restrictions on membership in the American Nurses' Association, which allowed African-American nurses to join only in 1950 (Carnegie, 1988; Hine, 1989).

Another challenge to biological theories of race is proposed by Fields (1990), who treats such theories as ideologies of race. Ideology is sometimes thought of as merely an idea, which can simply be substituted with new ideas through reeducation when the first idea proves ineffective or incorrect. Fields maintains that ideologies about race are legally sanctioned, reinforced through routinization, and inscribed upon the body of the individual. Both the repetition and carrying out of that idea over time are necessary. Without sanctions and regular practice, the idea dies. She uses the example of the enslavement of Africans and African Americans as paradigmatic of the ideology of race in America. A myriad of micropractices, carried out over the time and space of one's life, serve to remind us of our embodied state as legal property or as legal property owner, and consequences of life as raced individuals. Guillaumin (1988) points out that a previously circumstantial association of skin color and economic status can become its own evidence and justification. Nature, spontaneous and permanent, provides the mark, skin color for example, justifying and naturalizing enslavement. The relations between people and the social work of re/producing race are obscured in our fascination with this mark.

Finally, I would like to propose that race, like gender, as de Lauretis (1987) has demonstrated, is also a representation not of particular individuals, but of social relations among persons. I have argued that race is not a property of bodies, nor originally extant in human beings. Instead, race is a set of effects produced in bodies. The body is the site of technological interventions, not a raw material, which when examined gives up its secrets of race. Someone's race is usually considered self-evident, not found out in a lab test (yet?). The system of race, like and in cooperation with systems of gender, is what de Lauretis calls a "semiotic apparatus"—a system for assigning meaning and value to individuals within society. As such, the individual is both represented by and represents the self.

I have spoken of marks, micropractices, routinization, and the re/production of race as work. All of these are aspects of the technologies of race. What do I mean by these terms, and how do they interrelate?

Each of us has by now probably had many opportunities in which to indicate racial/ethnic origin in educational, employment, and census forms. Determination of these preordained categories and formalized rules for categorizing respondents is part of the work of the re/production of race. Checking the boxes is a routinized micropractice. The "work" of these activities becomes obvious when racially/ethnically ambiguous subjects confront the categories. What if the subject has parents from groups identified on the form as racially different? Should one check the box one most "looks" like? This might involve "marks" such as eye shape and skin and eye color, and might vary depending on the origins of the persons doing the looking. Some states still have legal standards categorizing, for example, persons of 1/32 African-American ancestry as black, appearances aside (Omi & Winant, 1986).

The U.S. Department of Health Statistics (Cooper & David, 1986) categorizes all persons with two white parents as white, but if one parent is white and the other is not, the progeny is not white, but whatever the "other" category is. Children of black fathers are mostly considered black, but children of black mothers usually are given their father's race.

During the 1990 census, the Census Bureau reported in an ongoing series in the *Washington Post* that some people seemed to think that they did not fit any of the rapidly expanding numbers of census categories, but the bureau knew better. Mixed-race people were simply assigned whatever race they listed first, even though they had checked other! So much for natural categories.

These systems for the determination of race are all used to assign meaning to biographical and social experiences. They both reflect and reproduce the practices they supposedly just "record."

FOUR PROBLEMS IN PREVIOUS RESEARCH ON RACE AND HEALTH

In the previous pages, I have argued for the denaturalization of race and the denaturalization of the relationship between race and health. Nevertheless, technologies of race (e.g., segregation and classification) have had some very material consequences upon health research and on the health status of American people. I have identified four problematic representations of people of color in biomedical and nursing health research: (1) not present, (2) depersonalized objects of experimentation, (3) race/ethnicity as disease, and (4) study of culture without context. I have assumed that, in almost all cases, this research was done in good faith. An important point of this paper is that one's theory, language, and practices may be at odds with one's research on race and health. This is not meant as an inclusive review of all research on race and health, but as an examination of recurring problems and the beginning of a guide with which to critically examine such research.

Not Present

A critical examination of most biomedical and nursing journals reveals a dismaying preponderance of studies that list "convenience" samples of 90 to 100 percent "caucasians," unless, of course, studying the effects of race on health is the point of the study, despite the fact that the same diseases that kill caucasians also kill noncaucasians. White, European Americans are represented as raceless, cultureless, uniform, and homogeneous—the norm.

I have heard many reasons for using completely European-American samples, including: such people are "more articulate"; they don't have "cultural barriers"; we need a specific reason to study non-European Americans or otherwise we have to assume all groups are the same; and we need to have a normative (white) sample first, so we can compare them to other groups.

I have also heard that "those people don't want to talk to us." This, of course, assumes that the "don't" is their problem—"they" do not want to participate in research that "we" decided they needed in the first place. Perhaps the problem resides instead with the researchers, who may not have adequately educated themselves about the communities they wish to study. Does the research address the needs of the people, as the people have defined them? What benefits will come to the community as a result of participating in this research?

Instead of relying entirely upon what biomedical scientists have said about populations that they wish to study, some researchers, including nurses, have taken time to study and become known in these communities, not just concerning themselves with the diseases that affect them. Jo Ann Banks-Wallace and Ama Saran, colleagues of mine at the University of Washington and themselves African-American women, have begun a local project to use focus groups to ask African-American women what sorts of research they would like to participate in and what sorts of health information these women think they need. Reading the literature produced by the people of interest about their own concerns is also often helpful (see, for example, White, 1990).

Race/Ethnicity as Source of Disease

Some of the worst abuses of people in the name of science and the promotion of the health of a nation, of course, occurred within German medicine under the Nazis. Less well known is the extent of Nazi medicine's borrowing of ideology from North American eugenicists in the 1930s and the degree to which biomedical science was utilized in providing the rationale and the technology for killing as a means of "racial hygiene" (Lifton, 1986). Lifton argues that medicine under the Nazis was not so much an aberration as an example of the ways in which the language, value system, and practices of biomedicine can, under the right circumstances, be called into the service of genocide. His analysis demonstrates the complex ideology and infrastructure needed to conduct a medicalized genocide on such a large scale.

Lifton points out that early difficulties with the psychological and physical decompensation in significant numbers of those called upon to do the actual killing necessitated the reconceptualization of killing as a "therapeutic imperative" (p. 15); that is, growing numbers of workers suffered physical and mental illness when called upon to hurt and kill. In order to ensure continuing participation, tasks related to killing were bureaucratized, or split into incremental pieces (micropractices) and dispersed over a greater number of people, so that any one person was usually responsible for one part in an entire chain of actions. These actions were then united under the ideology of hygiene.

Hitler reconceptualized post-World War I German demoralization as a disease and, taking advantage of long-standing, institutionalized prejudice against Jews, made the elimination of Jews and racial impurity in general the solution to the problems of the state. Jews, along with Africans, had long been associated with syphilis, then a most stigmatizing and devastating incurable disease. The "facts" of race, determined by skin color in Africans and the shape of the nose in Jews, were associated with a special propensity toward becoming syphilitic, despite the empirical fact that syphilis was a serious health problem for many, regardless of race. The cause of disease in the body, like the dis-ease of the state, was considered somehow inborn, both the result and a confirmation of one's problematic race.

A more modern example of race as source of disease is Rushton and Bogaert's (1989) controversial article about AIDS incidence. They propose that the higher incidence of AIDS in what they term "negroid" peoples of African ancestry is a natural evolutionary consequence in the form of population differences in "sexual restraint." Thus, increased incidence of AIDS is explained by genetics, as an "uninhibited disorder such as rape and unintended pregnancy" (p. 1211). Similarly, they proposed genetic, evolution-based reasons for greater frequency of low sexual excitement, premature ejaculation, and less sexually transmitted disease in peoples of Asian ancestry (relative to caucasians).

Leslie (1990), among others, has provided a rebuttal in which he points out the poor science, complete lack of regard for the consideration of environmental factors, and circularity of the arguments presented by Rushton and Bogaert. The homogeneity, heirarchy, and separate evolution of three races is itself an outdated and much discredited topic. Yet Rushton and Bogaert use the fact of differences in AIDS rates as both proof of the very existence of races themselves and of the genetic inferiority of very diverse groups of people. That more people of African descent around the world have HIV/AIDS at this time is not under dispute, however; the causal hypothesis is. Leslie points out that the surface "truth value" of the paper is enhanced by aspects of the structuring of the arguments, assumptions, and appearance of the paper, and of the appeals to "common sense" understandings about race likely to be held among the (assumed audience of white, Western male) scientists likely to read the paper. Rushton and Bogaert are, of course, appealing to the "natural" and to the "objectivity" of bodies in their explanations of AIDS incidence, as if this were de facto proof of the truth of their causal hypotheses and a castigation of Leslie for acknowledging his own feelings, his own history, and the history of race in anthropology in his understandings of the problem.

Objects of Experimentation

The U.S. Tuskegee syphilis experiment, which began at about the same time as the "racial hygiene" of the Nazis in the 1930s and continued until 1975, is still defended as "good science" even today. Under Tuskegee, low-income exclusively African-American men were invited to "participate" in a health study, in return for which they would receive some health care, treatment (a placebo), and a burial plot. The men were recruited and monitored by an African-American nurse who served to provide human contact and support to increase the likelihood that the men would remain in the study. The participants were not informed that this was a study about the long-term effects of untreated syphilis. Effective treatment was actively withheld and even prevented long after it was developed and widely available to the general public. During the 1970s, the U.S. Public Health Service debated the "deleterious" effects to the study of finally treating the men with penicillin. Finally, in 1973, the government began the task of locating the surviving men and arranging to treat them and to provide lifelong medical coverage to them.

Despite the initial good intentions of the researchers involved in this study, who appeared genuinely concerned with the health of African Americans and interested in eliminating syphilis, the researchers seemed uninterested in the eventual questions and protests of scientists and others that this study was of questionable benefit. A longer study, they argued, would provide more knowledge for the benefit of mankind, even at the cost of the suffering and reduced longevity of the individual subjects. Such suffering of individuals was worthwhile, as the group would benefit. Besides, many of the subjects were at such an advanced state that the use of penicillin was considered "deleterious" to them, or at least unhelpful. Treatment remained a "medical," not an ethical, question.

While some of these scientists professed horror at the atrocities of the Nazi doctors, the Tuskegee doctors saw themselves as just doing their jobs, ignoring the fact that what they were doing was, among other things, against even Alabama law.

Finally, a Czechoslovakian-born social worker, Public Health Service investigator Peter Buxton (who had fled with his family the Nazi occupation of his birthplace), enlisted the aid of the press in order to expose the abuses of Tuskegee to the general American and world public, which in turn lead to the end of the study and to some compensation for its subjects. Despite assurances to the contrary, none of the knowledge from the study will ever "prevent, find, or cure a single case" of syphilis.

Many questions remain, among them, why were African Americans and not wealthy European Americans chosen to be the subjects of this study? Why was vital information withheld for so long from the study participants? Jones (1981) speculates that the relative social and physical distance between researchers and subjects contributed to the researchers' lack of regard for the subjects as fully human beings like themselves. The use of an intermediary who was of lower status, who had no part in formulating the research questions, design, and procedures, and who was operating with limited information about the study is also questionable.

While present concerns about human subject protection render the chances for such experiments relatively remote, I am still left with questions. Where are the ethics of providing opportunities for health care services within research studies for persons for which other health care opportunities are limited? When conducting research on military and incarcerated populations, is consent fully informed and freely given? Considering the overrepresentation of people of color in such populations, are people of color also overrepresented in these types of studies? To what degree do we, in our present studies, continue to use people of color as intermediaries, ill informed, with little input, and serving as the means to access communities?

Culture without Context

Taussig (1992) has emphasized the importance of considering context in conducting and thinking about research, remembering that researchers themselves are part of that context. One's own values, beliefs, culture, and experiences certainly affect not only one's research, but one's practice, teaching, and other scholarship as well. We are sometimes tempted to try to put aside our contexts, but I am convinced that the assumptions we're not aware of can be the most problematic.

Chrisman (1991) notes that, to many of us, culture is something someone else has. We are then tempted to go study this "other" in its pristine, unchanging separateness, not considering that we are also bringing our own changing selves and cultures into the interaction or that we, too, are being studied. We might think we're leaving our preconceived notions behind, and yet our interactions with this "other" are continually being informed by our previous understandings, just as the "other's" impressions are similarly informed by preconceived notions, understandings, and history. Why do we imagine ourselves invisible or imagine that the "other" is seeing us as we'd like to be seen: benevolent, wise, powerful, and kind?

A few years ago, I attended a regional nursing research conference in which a symposium of ethnographic research studies was presented. During the discussion, I raised a question that has long concerned me: how to avoid exploiting the very vulnerable populations that all of us were studying and trying to help. Good intentions, unfortunately, are not enough, and I wondered if that question might not be sometimes on the minds of study participants.

One of the presentations was an interesting study on reasons for noncompliance with treatment in endstage diabetic men of a certain Native-American tribe. The researchers seemed to be looking for incongruence between traditional and Western biomedical health and illness beliefs, itself a very important question. However, while accessibility of care was explored, the context of the delivery of care, of reservation life, and of the relations between the tribe and nontribal (white) persons did not seem to come under consideration. In the interest of fairness, I emphasized the brevity of the time provided, even as I wondered what kinds of issues were deemed more important when time, resources, and money remain scarce.

Researchers may not see themselves in terms of race. Yet I wondered what the men in the diabetes study saw, whose tribe was participating in a continuing land rights dispute with a predominantly white government and neighbors, simultaneously receiving care from a health care system similarly influenced, and talking to a white researcher from a state institution. Would I have trusted the health care providers or the researcher? What do they know about me, and what do they think there is to know?

The point is not that only Native Americans can study Native Americans and so on, but that, as demonstrated by the Swinomish Tribes' (1991) publication on tribal mental health, a sense of the history and context of a people, informed by that people, is necessary. Included within this context is some knowledge of the relationships between the people and the researcher/practitioner/educator and their various ethnic, institutional, and other pertinent reference groups.

Consequences for Health Research

I have watched changes in health policy and practices related to "race" with some interest. I have noticed a fairly continuous lack of awareness and commitment to understanding and questioning the discourse on race in nursing, though I remain hopeful about present attempts to correct this. It is my contention that members of ethnic minority groups, or "people of color," a term preferred by some because it denotes coalition among groups differentiated by racial discourse, have with good reason considerable suspicion about this newly discovered interest within NIH.

The absence of research is, of course, a starting place. The silences are part of the discourse on race and health, products of the historical, sociopolitical, and symbolic environments influencing the production of health care research. Where are the silences, and why those particular silences? In what ways does health care research reflect the dominant cultural view of persons of color? But before we seek to "fill" these silences, we need to understand them, their meaning, and their significance. Simply extracting more information about "race" from individuals may not be helpful; it may extend the problem. I have sought to examine the discourse on race and on race and health, asking not what is race but with a brief description of discourse. The problem arises in "naturalizing" discourses on race within the theory and practices of nursing and health research. I offer this paper with the interest of producing better quality health care for all and in promoting a greater sense of responsibility and accountability in health care researchers.

DISCUSSION QUESTIONS

1. Allman distinguishes "discourse on race" from "race." What does she mean by this difference and why is it important?

2. According to Allman, what happens when discourses, such as those on race or gender, are "naturalized" or made into "scientific" discourses? What are the consequences?

3. Allman and Thompson both raise questions about the "problem" of theorizing. A similar concern is raised by Hiraki. Using "race" or another concept of your choosing (including perhaps, "nursing"), discuss the potentially negative consequences of developing theories about "race" or "nursing" and how these consequences might be addressed.

REFERENCES

Carnegie, M. E. (1988). In T. M. Schoor & A. Simmerman (Eds.), *Making choices taking chances* (pp. 28–42). St. Louis: C. V. Mosby.

Chrisman, N. J. (1991). Ethnic persistence in an urban setting. *Ethnicity, 8*, 256–292.

Cooper, R., & David, R. (1986). The biological concept of race and its application to public health and epidemiology. *Journal of Health Politics, Policy & Law, 11*(1), 97–116.

de Lauretis, T. (1987). *Technologies of gender*. Bloomington: Indiana University Press.

Dreyfus, H. L., & Rabinow, P. (1982/83). *Michel Foucault: Beyond structuralism and hermeneutics* (2nd ed.). Chicago: University of Chicago Press.

Fields, B. (1990). Racism in America. *New Left Review, 181*, 95–118.

Foucault, M. (1977). In D. F. Bouchard (Ed.), *Michel Foucault: Language, countermemory and practice*. New York: Cornell University.

Foucault, M. (1982/83). The subject and power. In H. L. Dreyfus & P. Rabinow (Eds.). *Michel Foucault: Beyond structuralism and hermeneutics* (2nd ed.). Chicago: University of Chicago Press.

Funkhouser, S. H., & Moser, D. K. (1990). Is health care racist? *Advances in Nursing Science, 12*(2), 47–55.

Gilman, S. (1991). *The Jew's body*. New York: Routledge.

Gordon, D. R. (1988). Tenacious assumptions in western medicine. In M. Lock & D. Gordon (Eds.), *Biomedicine examined*. Boston: Kluwer.

Guillaumin, C. (1988). Race and nature: The system of marks. The idea of a natural group and social relationships (M. J. Lakeland, Trans.). *Feminist Issues, 8*(2), 25–43.

Haraway, D. (1988). Situated knowledges: The science question in feminism and the privilege of partial perspective. *Feminist Studies, 14*(3), 575–599.

Haraway, D. (1992). The promises of monsters: A regenerative politics for inappropriate/d others. In L. Grossberg, C. Nelson, & P. Treichler (Eds.), *Cultural studies* (pp. 295–337). New York: Routledge.

Hine, D. C. (1989). *Black women in white: Racial conflict and cooperation in the nursing profession, 1890–1950*. Bloomington: Indiana University Press.

Jones, J. H. (1981). *Bad blood: the Tuskegee syphilis experiment—A tragedy of race and medicine*. New York: Basic Books.

Leslie, C. (1990). Scientific racism: Reflections on peer review, science and ideology. *Social Science & Medicine, 31*(3), 891–905.

Lifton, R. J. (1986). *Nazi doctors: Medical killing and the psychology of genocide.* New York: Basic Books.

National Institutes of Health. (1990). *NIH Guide 19*(38), 1–10.

Omi, M., & Winant, H. (1986). *Racial formation in the United States: From the 1960s to the 1980s.* New York: Routledge & Kegal Paul.

Polednak, A. P. (1989). *Racial and ethnic differences in disease.* New York: Oxford University Press.

Rushton, J. P. (1990). Comments on scientific racism. *Social Science & Medicine, 31*(3), 905–909.

Rushton, J. P., & Bogaert, A. F. (1989). Population differences in susceptibility to AIDS: An evolutionary analysis. *Social Science & Medicine, 28*(12), 1211–1220.

Swinomish Tribal Mental Health Project (1991). *A gathering of wisdoms.* La Conner, WA: Swinomish Tribal Community.

Taussig, M. (1992). *The nervous system.* New York: Routledge.

White, E. C. (1990). *The black women's health book: Speaking for ourselves.* Seattle: Seal Press.

Winant, H. (1990). Postmodern racial politics: Difference and inequality. *Socialist Review, 46/7*, 121–147.

Yamato, G. (1990). Something about the subject makes it hard to name. In G. Anzaldua (Ed.), *Making face, making soul haciendo caras* (pp. 20–24). San Francisco: Aunt Lute Foundation.

4

Eve's Legacy: An Analysis of Family Caregiving from a Feminist Perspective

Sheila M. Bunting

*I*n the biblical book of *Genesis*, just after Eve had tasted the apple, shared it with Adam, made her first dress out of leaves, and been scolded and expelled from paradise by God, we find the verse: *"The man called his wife's name Eve, because she was the mother of all living."* "Eve" comes from a Hebrew word meaning "mother." At that point, according to the traditional Bible (the gnostic gospels tell another story), motherhood and the caregiving associated with it began.

Where will it all end?

The author gratefully acknowledges the assistance of Dr. Jacquelyn Campbell for her critical reading and suggestions on a previous draft of this paper.

Research leading to the writing of this paper was supported by predoctoral student awards from the National Center for Nursing Research (5 F31 NR06440-02) and from the Michigan Health Care Education and Research Foundation, the research and philanthropic affiliate of Blue Cross and Blue Shield of Michigan (067-SAP/91-08).

INTRODUCTION

The care given by family and friends to those who are unable to care for themselves has long been an important focus for nursing theory, practice, and research. The conflicts and health concerns of caregivers (Bunting, 1989; Robinson, 1988) as well as caregiver strategies (Bowers, 1987; Phillips & Rempusheski, 1986) have been the subject of empirical, ethical, and theoretical nursing inquiry. In the United States, the primary goal of many of these studies has been the support of the caregivers (frequently women) to enable them to continue the caregiving process. The financial benefits for the national economy and the humane interests of the care receiver have often been cited as important outcomes of keeping caregiving in the home. Most discussions have centered on the microsystem of the caregiver/care receiver dyad or on the immediate family providing care (O'Neill & Sorensen, 1991). The need for study of any single aspect of health care within the context of the historical, social, and other influences in which it occurs has been recognized by feminist theorists (Reverby, 1987; Tronto, 1987) and nurses (Allen, Benner, & Diekelmann, 1986; Anderson, 1990; Hedin, 1989; Stevens, 1989; Thompson, 1987) and is a basic premise of the social critical theory and feminist research methodologies. This article will take the framework used by Hare-Mustin (1988) in conceptualizing the separation between the private and public social spheres and apply it to the caregiver situation to expand extant nursing views of this important construct.

CAREGIVING AS A WOMEN'S ISSUE

In nearly every area of practice, nurses have been made aware that family caregiving, particularly caregiving to the frail elderly, is a women's issue: both the caregiver and the care receiver are likely to be women. The professional caregivers—nurses and social workers who provide and coordinate services for the families—are also likely to be women, and the attitudes of these professionals have a major impact on family caregiving. In this paper, therefore, I will examine and discuss the origins of attitudes toward caregiving which may prevail among nurses as well as in society at large. For instance, nurses may assume that care in the home by a woman relative is better and more cost-effective than professional care. Nursing research and practice may be aimed at keeping the caregiver caring, whatever the personal cost in the caregiver's own life.

In addition, I will critique the ideology of family caregiving from a feminist and critical theory perspective. Also considered are the associated social and political expectations and the policies which are consequences of the ideology of caregiving.

Ubiquity of Female Caregiving

In these times of increasing longevity, women may spend their entire lives giving care. They provide this care to various recipients in different ways throughout their life spans, beginning with baby-sitting their siblings, continuing by caring for their own children, their aged parents and other relatives, and often ending with caring for their debilitated husbands. Caring is taught, modeled, and rewarded as a moral ideal to little girls, and until recent decades, "caring" professions such as nursing, social work, and teaching were seen as those most appropriate for women.

Definition of Caregiving

For this paper, informal caregiving is broadly conceptualized as a process of taking responsibility for and providing for the needs of another, including emotional, social, spiritual, and other needs as well as the physical. They include maintenance of the environment of the care receiver—such needs do emerge as variables in the caregiver literature. Actions, thoughts, and feelings of the one caring may be considered a part of caregiving. As a result, caregiving may be burdensome for both giver and receiver and may lead to strained relations between them (Orem, 1991). It may also be pleasant and satisfying at times, which is not to say it is not a responsibility, taking energy and time.

Ideology of Caregiving

Leininger (1988) and the many nurses supporting her theory of Culture Care Diversity with their transcultural studies on care have demonstrated that care and caregiving are universals. For all peoples, care is a necessary condition for the maintenance of human existence.

The ideologies of care, however, may be culture specific. Pope, Quinn, and Wyer (1990) said that the fantasy of the perfect mother, which is the prototype of caregiving, is a product of the patriarchal Western ideal of the nuclear family. The myth turns out to be stronger than the reality; when women's experience of mothering is different from the myth, they assume their experience is false, rather than questioning the myth. As Pope, Quinn, and Wyer point out, "in the collision of reality with mythology, it is the mythology that tends to prevail" (p. 445). The idealization of caregiving, as a strategy to perpetuate the patriarchal myth, supports the ideology that woman is the sole provider for the emotional and physical care needs of the family and, by extension, of society.

Women as "Natural Caregivers"

Women are often seen as being "natural" caregivers—as having a gift for meeting the needs of others by the very fact that they are women. From a functionalist perspective, it is easy to assume that, because women's bodies are equipped to gestate and provide nutrition for offspring, women are genetically programmed or socially or divinely decreed to care for others. Like so many self-fulfilling prophesies, this also comes true: more women than men are caregivers—daughters, daughters-in-law, sisters, mothers, and granddaughters.

In her illuminating book *Women in the Middle*, Brody (1989) pointed out: "My two brothers and I are attorneys. When our mother, who lives in Florida, fractured a hip, everyone assumed that I would fly down and stay for a while. My brothers are good sons, but my suggestion that we take turns met with surprise. They said they had 'to earn a living'" (p. ix).

Alpha Bias and Beta Bias

Rachel Hare-Mustin (1988), a feminist professor of counseling and human relations at Villanova University, has addressed the idea of the so-called "natural" gender differences between women and men. She points out that the isolating, or dichotomizing, of phenomena is a customary method of analyzing anything under study, especially by scientists. This method is also used by many of those feminists, sometimes labeled "cultural feminists" (Bunting & Campbell, 1990; Hoffman, 1991), who hold the position that women are inherently or culturally different (i.e., better) than men. In the case of the relationships between men and women, Hare-Mustin (1988) believes that this dicohtomy has led to a false emphasis on female and male as opposites—an exaggeration of differences rather than a recognition of commonalities. Hare-Mustin characterized this emphasis as a bias, a systematic inclination to emphasize certain experiences and overlook others. She labeled the exaggeration of differences between groups such as women and men "alpha" bias. The minimizing of differences which actually do exist (such as the greater need of a mother than a father to recover from childbirth) was termed "beta" bias. Examples of alpha bias in social theories include the sex role theory of Parsons and Bales (1955) as well as theories which emphasize developmental differences between genders, including the theories of Erikson (1968), Chodorow (1974), and Gilligan (1982).

Sex role theory is a part of structural functionalist theory based on the concept that social structures have developed in response to the needs of the members of a given society. In this theory, relationships and roles of individuals serve a purpose or function in maintaining the society (i.e., the woman's roles as child caretaker and homemaker not only promote the "good" of the society, but are necessary for its maintenance). Theories of developmental difference hold that male and female children develop along different courses, either because of the psychological responses to genital differences or to the differences in their relationships with their mothers.

Women Socialized into Caregiving Mode

The functional theory of women's "natural" proclivity to care gains credence from the fact that women have been culturally and socially encouraged to value care. Women do demonstrate a valuing of care in the priorities they have established in their personal and social lives. They feel responsible *to* others and *for* others. While not restricted to women, feelings and behaviors associated with taking responsibility for others' well-being is more pronounced in women, and women are more likely to feel guilt for what *might* have been done (Horowitz, 1985).

Although responsibility and caring are desirable and socially beneficial, a problem arises from the fact that there are larger and larger numbers of elderly and others with chronic illness who are not able to care for themselves and who must therefore be cared for by someone. In a disproportionate number of cases that someone is a woman carrying care responsibility alone.

Private vs. Public Spheres: Historical Perspective

Many feminist analysts (Chow & Berheide, 1988; Hare-Mustin, 1988; Hooyman, 1990; Ryan, 1987) who attempt to explain the present situation of caregiving conceptualize it as tied to the status of women's work within the private sector. In earlier times, many of life's necessities, such as food, clothing, medicines, and household goods, were produced within the family environment or bartered for with such home-produced goods. Such conditions are termed "preindustrial" in the sense of having occurred in a time or place before large percentages of household and other goods were manufactured in mechanized and organized factories.

Before the time of large-scale organized production of goods outside the home, the contributions of women to the ongoing survival and functioning of the tribe was as important as that of men, though women's work was less valued in most societies (e.g., if hunting was done by men, meat was more valued even if the roots and tubers provided by the women were a more vital part of the diet) (Friedl, 1975; O'Kelly & Carney, 1986). In preindustrial societies the contributions of women did receive recognition; social thinking did not make a separation between work associated with family maintenance and work associated with production of other goods.

In modern times, however, the family is not the primary unit of production and family welfare is governed by a wage economy. This has resulted in a separation of household production from paid work. Because women receive no wages for the labor performed in their homes, they are in the position of performing services and producing products for the family that have no recognized market value (Hare-Mustin, 1988). This situation has added to the devalued status of women in the home and in society, because in the present socioeconomic situation one is valued according to what one is paid. Adding to this problem is the fact that social scientists and historians, in analyzing industrialized societies, recorded chiefly the activities of men. For the most part, they overlooked contributions of women, children, and old people who did not earn a wage (Hare-Mustin, 1988).

Household Production as Valuable

According to Hare-Mustin (1988) the emphasis on industrial production outside the home has led people to act as though the home no longer produces anything important, and this is not true. Whereas households may no longer produce goods for sale, certainly these settings produce meals, clean laundry, and shelter for the masses. Surely homes are collectively *the* largest service industry, at least in the United States, where women coordinate the social-ization, education, health care, purchasing, and waste control of the majority of the population. Despite their increased likelihood to be working outside the home, middle-class mothers, by use of the automobile, provide trans-portation of goods and people at a rate which is mind-boggling. Hare-Mustin (1988) concludes that "What modern technology has done is allow the housewife to produce by herself and at a higher standard what had required the services of other family members in the past" (p. 37).

Effects of Separation of Public vs. Private

The separation of the public sphere of the work place and the private sphere of the home was perpetuated in the late nineteenth and early twentieth centuries by legislation and unions as well as by company policies that banned nepotism and the participation of women in the work place. Workers were discouraged from the intermingling of work and family life because industrial management did not want family problems to interfere with productivity (Chow & Berheide, 1988). The home became idealized as a haven where the breadwinning man could recuperate from the stresses of the competitive work environment (Hare-Mustin, 1988; Ryan, 1987). This idealization of the home as a haven has also had long-range effects on the view of the proper setting for caregiving.

Influx of Women to the Work Place

Whereas many poor women have always worked for pay outside of the home, a dramatic change in the twentieth century has been the influx of middle-class wives into the paid work force. Between 1960 and 1985 alone, the participation rate for married women with children under 18 rose from 28 to 61 percent (Taeuber & Valdisera, 1986). Despite this increased par-ticipation of women in the paid work force, a demand which was added to their home responsibilities, the research that has been done on work-related stress has focused largely on men. This may possibly reflect a male view that women's roles in the home are somehow "natural" and therefore do not induce stress. It may also reflect the view that because most women are employed in sex-segregated and low paying jobs, their work-related stress should be less than that of men.

Semipermeable Boundaries

The boundaries between the work and family spheres are not symmetrical; they are semipermeable membranes for both men and women—but in different directions. For women, the lack of support for the care of the myriad needs of children, dependent adults, and the home itself means that their home responsibilities (e.g., appliance repair, someone to let the plumber in) intrude into the work domain. For men, the membrane permeability goes in the other direction in that it is usually acceptable for men to bring business work home. They may also use family time to recover from occupationally-induced stress (e.g., "Please give me half-an-hour to unwind before you confront me with problems with the children.").

Caregiving as Invisible Work

Caregiving by women to family members is invisible in the sense that it is not counted in the calculations of the national or family economy. Similarly to housework, which is only noticed when it is *not* provided, there is an assumption that caregiving will somehow be provided by the family, and "family" is all too often a euphemism for one female relative.

Ward (1987, 1990) did a secondary analysis on data collected in a large randomized national survey (Stone, Cafferata, & Sangle, 1987) to study the economic implications of the work of caregiving. She likened what she termed "kin care" to housework (Hartmann, 1981), which is invisible because it is unpaid labor. Such work is considered "free" by a society that undervalues work provided by women in the private sector. Ward (1990) pointed out that "home care is less costly than hospital care only when kin care is assigned no value" (p. 230).

Both Ward (1990) and Colliere (1986), a French nurse who has written on "invisible" caregiving, identified the theoretical and historical connections between the devaluing of women's care in the home and the difficulty of gaining recognition for *nurses'* contributions of care. There is a relationship between the lack of prestige and respect for caregiving in the private sphere of the home and the low status of nursing as a profession. Both nursing and caregiving are examples of the invisibility of care related to the blurring of the boundaries between the public and private sectors. In the public sector, work is recognized, valued, and paid for, whereas in the private sector, work is treated as a labor of love or duty.

This ambiguity of the public and private aspects of caring work was also noted by Gibeau (1986), who studied the effects of the caregiving work of daughters and daughters-in-law on their paid employment and their personal lives. She found that the combined average hours per week of kin care and housework was 35, nearly the equivalent of a second full-time job. It would be interesting to calculate what this would cost in wages if the services were provided by an agency, but the resulting figure would still not include the losses women take in giving up promotions and overtime wages in their paying jobs. This forgoing of promotions and lack of investment in their careers places women at a disadvantage in their retirement, leaving them more vulnerable to poverty and more likely to need unpaid care from their own daughters.

Gibeau (1986) found that employed women caregivers who spent fewer contact hours in actual care were those who used income from their paid work to pay other women to care for their disabled elders. This provides another example of the ambiguity of the economy of private sector care.

Ryan (1987), in her interviews with caseworkers of the elderly, found that these workers, primarily women and underpaid professional caregivers themselves, believed care in the home by a loved one was superior to agency care. They considered the well-being of the care receiver to be more important than that of the caregiver. The fact that a majority (68 percent) of these professionals thought of caregiver welfare as a secondary consideration is significant for its probable effect on funding and policy decisions. Such an expectation supports the myth and ideology of the ideal of woman-provided care in the home. The attitude definitely affects the perceptions and feelings of the caregivers.

Hooyman (1990) used the term "new conservatism" to refer to the emphasis on fiscal restraints, cost effectiveness, efficiency, and privatization of family responsibilities that became more pronounced during the 1980s. There is an increasing value placed on moving the elderly and the disabled, including the chronically mentally ill, out of institutions. This ideology of community care, which favors keeping such individuals in their own communities, has had major effects on deinstitutionalization policies (Briar & Ryan, 1986). The new conservatism, combined with the ideology of community care, has had a double effect: it increases the inequality of family caregiving as it increases the burden. The new conservatism described by Hooyman (1990) promoted the idea that uncompensated care in the community is more humane, sensitive, and superior in every way to professional care. Such a notion is also based on the assumption that someone in that home is able and can be persuaded or coerced to make the necessary life changes to provide the care.

The assumption (Ward, 1990) that caregiving in the home given by women is free underlies much of the public policy and the research which has proliferated on the topic of caregiving. Home caregiving is conceptualized as an untapped national resource that should be better utilized. If caregivers are experiencing burden and strain, the research often addresses the question of how these problems can be combated so that women can *continue to care*. A recent commentary (Bowers, 1990) on a nursing study of caregiver burden (Bull, 1990) cited as benefits of caregiver research the possibility that costs of care and elder abuse would be reduced. While decreased morbidity of the caregiver was mentioned, this advantage was treated as a secondary gain. This focus by nurses on the recipient of care to the neglect of the caregiver tends to represent caregivers as a means to an end. That end is the positive outcome of decreased cost of elder care.

It may not be immediately apparent that when policy makers and legislators attempt to promote family caregiving for cost savings, they are actually advocating that the private sector (women in the home) take over a responsibility that belongs to the larger society. Without women who put aside their own life goals and actually jeopardize their own futures to provide care, the number of elders in institutions would be tripled (Brody, 1981, 1989) and the estimated cost of kin care would amount to nearly $18 billion (Ward, 1990). Despite the ideology exemplified in the American ideal of taking care of "our own," the United States is one of the few industrialized nations that does not uniformly provide a stipend to family caregivers of the elderly, although many state programs do provide this support (Hooyman, 1990).

Ethnocentric and Androcentric Bias?

A feminist analysis of the research approaches to any issue includes the question of possible ethnocentric and androcentric bias (Campbell & Bunting, 1991). Ethnocentric bias can be noted in most caregiver literature in the fact that "subjects" of most published research are not categorized according to ethnicity. The ethnic background of the researchers cannot be known, although these are usually academia-based sociologists or gerontologists. In most reports it was apparent that values, concerns, and stressors such as strain or burden were presumed to be universal to all cultures—a very large presumption. Although the feminist research principles position investigators to document procedures for validating conclusions with informants (Duffy & Hedin, 1988), this was usually not done in reports of caregiver studies in the literature.

In general, the massive research on the topic of family caregiving is sympathetic to caregivers, and androcentric bias in studies may not be immediately apparent, given the early attention to the women's role in caregiving (Brody, 1981). There is, however, a gender-based division of labor in caregiving; men (other than spouses) tend to withdraw from the caregiving role when the condition of the elder causes caregiving demands to include housework and personal care (Stoller, 1990). There is an implicit perception of the female caregiver as a victim, self-sacrificing and overwhelmed with stress, rather than as a competent and self-sufficient achiever who manages caregiving with effective, often ingenious strategies. Whereas the relatively few sons who are caregivers are often perceived as heroes by relatives and neighbors (Horowitz, 1985), women caregivers are often regarded with pity and condescension. This perception may be related to the notion that men, particularly sons of disabled elderly, have choices about taking on the role of caregiver. The assumption may exist that women relatives, on the other hand, have an inherent duty to provide care for family members. This expectation of women engaging in caregiving was found to be dominant in the attitudes of professionals coordinating care for the elderly in Ryan's (1987) study discussed above. As nurses, we must question our own assumptions about families as we plan care.

CONCLUSION

Women take on the job of caregiving because they value care and the maintenance and nurturing of relationships (Gilligan, 1982) they consider essential for an acceptable quality of life. Many identify and feel connected with their mothers and therefore with others, taking on the caring role at an early age. The mother-daughter bond has been characterized as one of the most complicated, varied, and intense of human relationships (Boyd, 1990; Chodorow, 1978). Phillips and Rempusheski (1986), in a study of good and poor caregiving, found that identification of caregiver with care receiver was strongly related to higher quality caregiving of the elderly.

Daughters think about how their mothers took care of them, and they hope someone will care for them when they are old. They act out of love and duty and their belief that it is something that must be done by someone. They want the care of their own elders to be lovingly and compassionately given. But the responsibility for the care of the elderly needs to be better disbursed. As the baby-boomers reach old age, new ways of allocating caregiving must be discovered and put into use.

So what is the answer? It's not that women should quit caregiving. Caregiving is needed in our world more than it ever was in the past. A beginning move for nurses and other professional caregivers, as well as policy makers and legislators, is to examine their assumptions and expectations of caregivers and the caregiving experience. It is necessary to move beyond our alpha and beta biases; not all women are genetically superior caregivers, but those who do take on the role should not have to impoverish their present and future lives by surrendering their social contacts, their professional promotions, and their own self-care. Assistance to the growing population of elderly who need help is not the responsibility of a few relatives in the private sector, but of the community at large.

It is important for nurses to move beyond the microsystem in conceptualizing family/friend caregiving. Butterfield (1990) used the metaphor of health care providers continually pulling their clients from the rushing river of individual case management problems without the time or the vision to go upstream to find out what forces are pushing victims into the river. Using a critical social theory perspective which included structural and societal influences on the microsystem, Butterfield recommended that nurses engage in "upstream" thinking and action and that they take part in shaping policies for a change in the status quo. Such a metaphor would be appropriate for the family/friend caregiving situation in planning for a growing population of elderly.

The modern caregiver is not to be seen as a helpless victim, but as a hero, whether a woman or a man. In learning to integrate caregiving into their lives, caregivers have developed impressive resources and strategies. These successful managers have much to teach those of us who are professional caregivers. Not only can we pass on to our clients the survival skills we have learned from them, we can make use of these skills in our own lives. It is clear, in view of the caregiving statistics, that many nurses, women and men, will *be* caregivers in their personal as well as professional lives and will, it is hoped, receive care themselves when the time comes that such care is needed.

DISCUSSION QUESTIONS

1. This paper raises questions about the social construction of women's obligation to care. Bunting discusses this obligation both in terms of the sociohistorical development of capitalism and in terms of the subjectivity of women as caregivers. Why are both of these perspectives important?

2. In this paper, Bunting works from a feminist standpoint. Using her discussion of "alpha" and "beta" bias, discuss her analysis of women's obligation to care. Does she invite us to assume an alpha or a beta bias in our understanding of caregiving?

3. In comparing this paper with those of Gray, Henderson, and Hagell, what sort of feminist standpoint are we encouraged to assume? Comparing this paper with that of Allen, what are some of the intended consequences of focusing on gender as a category? What are some of the unintended consequences of focusing on gender as a category?

REFERENCES

Allen, D., Benner, P., & Diekelmann, N. L. (1986). Three paradigms for nursing research: Methodological implications. In P. Chinn (Ed.), *Nursing research methodology: Issues and implementation* (pp. 23–38). Rockville, MD: Aspen.

Anderson, J. M. (1990). Home care management in chronic illness and the self-care movement: An analysis of ideologies and economic processes influencing policy decisions. *Advances in Nursing Science, 12*(2), 71–83.

Bowers, B. J. (1987). Intergenerational caregiving: Adult caregivers and their aging parents. *Advances in Nursing Science, 9*(2), 20–32.

Bowers, J. E. (1990). Commentary. *Western Journal of Nursing Research, 12*(6), 771.

Boyd, C. (1990). Testing a model of mother-daughter identification. *Western Journal of Nursing Research, 12*(4), 448–468.

Briar, K., & Ryan, R. (1986). The anti-institution movement and women caregivers. *Affilia, 1*(1), 20–32.

Brody, E. M. (1981). Women in the middle and family help to older people. *The Gerontologist, 21*, 471–480.

Brody, E. M. (1989). *Women in the Middle.* New York: Springer.

Bull, M. J. (1990). Factors influencing family caregiver burden and health. *Western Journal of Nursing Research, 12*(6), 758–770.

Bunting, S. M. (1989). Stress on caregivers of the elderly. *Advances in Nursing Science, 11*(2), 63–73.

Bunting, S. M., & Campbell, J. C. (1990). Feminism and nursing: Historical perspectives. *Advances in Nursing Science, 12*(4), 11–24.

Butterfield, P. G. (1990). Thinking upstream: Nurturing a conceptual understanding of the societal context of health behavior. *Advances in Nursing Science, 12*(2), 1–8.

Campbell, J. C., & Bunting, S. M. (1991). Voices and paradigms: Perspectives on critical and feminist theory in nursing. *Advances in Nursing Science, 13*(3), 1–15.

Chodorow, N. (1974). Family structure and feminine personality. In M. Z. Rosaldo and L. Lamphere (Eds.), *Women, culture and society* (pp. 43–66). Stanford, CA: Stanford University Press.

Chodorow, N. (1978). *The reproduction of mothering: Psychoanalysis and the sociology of gender.* Berkeley: University of California Press.

Chow, E. N., & Berheide, C. W. (1988). The interdependence of family and work: A framework for family life education, policy, and practice. *Family Relations, 37*, 23–28.

Colliere, M. F. (1986). Invisible care and invisible women as health care providers. *International Journal of Nursing Studies, 23*(2), 95–112.

Duffy, M. & Hedin, B. A. (1988). New directions for nursing research. In N. F. Woods & M. Catanzaro (Eds.), *Nursing research: Theory and practice* (pp. 530–539). St. Louis: C. V. Mosby.

Erikson, E. H. (1968). *Identity, youth, and crisis.* New York: Norton

Friedl, E. (1975). *Women and men.* New York: Holt, Rinehart & Winston.

Gibeau, J. (1986). Breadwinners and caregivers: Working patterns of women working full-time and caring for dependent elderly family members (Doctoral dissertation), Brandeis University, Watham, MA.

Gilligan, C. (1982). *In a different voice.* Cambridge, MA: Harvard University Press.

Hare-Mustin, R. T. (1988). Family change and gender differences: Implications for theory and practice. *Family Relations, 37*, 36–41.

Hartmann, H. (1981). The family as the locus of gender, class, and political struggle: The example of housework. *Signs, 6*(3), 366–394.

Hedin, B. A. (1989). Nursing education and sterile ethical fields. *Advances in Nursing Science, 11*(3), 43–52.

Hoffman, F. (1991). Feminism and nursing, *NWSA Journal, 3*(1), 53–69.

Hooyman, N. R. (1990). Women as caregivers of the elderly: Implications for social welfare policy and practice. In D. E. Biegel & A. Blum (Eds.). *Aging and caregiving: Theory, research, and policy* (pp. 221–241). Newbury Park, CA: Sage.

Horowitz, A. (1985). Sons and daughters as caregivers to parents: Differences in role performance and consequences. *The Gerontologist, 25,* 612–617.

Leininger, M. M. (1988). Leininger's theory of nursing: Cultural care diversity and universality. *Nursing Science Quarterly, 1*(4), 152–160.

O'Kelly, C. G., & Carney, L. S. (1986). *Women and men in society: Cross-cultural perspectives on gender stratification.* Belmont, CA: Wadsworth.

O'Neill, C., & Sorensen, E. S. (1991). Home care of the elderly: A family perspective. *Advances in Nursing Science, 13*(4), 28–37.

Orem, D. E. (1991). *Nursing concepts of practice.* (4th ed.). St. Louis: C. V. Mosby.

Parsons, T., & Bales, R. F. (1955). *Family, socialization, and interaction process.* Glencoe, IL: Free Press.

Phillips, L. A., & Rempusheski, V. F. (1986). Caring for the frail elderly at home: Toward a theoretical explanation of the dynamics of poor quality family caregiving. *Advances in Nursing Science, 8*(4), 62–84.

Pope, D., Quinn, N., & Wyer, M. (1990). The ideology of mothering: Disruption and reproduction of patriarchy. *Signs, 15*(3), 441–446.

Reverby, S. M. (1987). *Ordered to care: The dilemma of American nursing, 1850–1945.* New York: Cambridge University Press.

Robinson, K. M. (1988). A social skills training program for adult caregivers. *Advances in Nursing Science, 10*(2), 59–72.

Ryan, R. (1987). Clients or service providers: How case managers view the relatives of frail elders (Doctoral dissertation, University of Washington). *Dissertation Abstracts International,* 8810588.

Stevens, P. E. (1989). A critical social reconceptualization of environment in nursing: Implications for methodology. *Advances in Nursing Science, 11*(4), 56–68.

Stoller, E. P. (1990). Males as helpers: The role of sons, relatives, and friends. *The Gerontologist, 30*(2), 228–235.

Stone, R., Cafferata, G. L., & Sangle, J. (1987). Caregivers of the frail elderly: A national profile. *The Gerontologist, 7,* 616–626.

Taeuber, C. M., & ValDisera, V. W. (1986). *Women in the American economy.* U.S. Bureau of the Census, Current Population Reports, Series P-32, No. 146. Washington, DC: U.S. Government Printing Office.

Thompson, J. L. (1987). Critical scholarship: The critique of domination in nursing. *Advances in Nursing Science, 10*(1), 27–38.

Tronto, J. C. (1987). Beyond gender difference to a theory of care. *Signs, 12*(4), 644–663.

Ward, D. H. (1987). The new old burden: Gender and cost in kin care of disabled elderly (Doctoral dissertation, Boston University). *Dissertation Abstracts International,* 8806498.

Ward, D. H. (1990). Gender, time, and money in caregiving. *Scholarly Inquiry for Nursing Practice, 4*(3), 223–234.

5

Nursing and the Caring Metaphor: Gender and Political Influences on an Ethics of Care

Esther H. Condon

*I*n this paper, I will explore gender and political influences on an ethics of care as they impact upon its relevance as an ethics for nursing. The following topics will be included in the discussion: the historical influence of gender upon the public influence of women; the division of labor along gender lines that has placed the responsibility for caring activities almost exclusively on women; current models of interpersonal caring of interest to nursing; examples of feminist critique of one of these models; an example of feminist philosophy that would support an ethics of caring for nursing; and conclusions concerning the relevance of an ethics of caring for nursing. In order to take any position about the relevance of an ethics of caring for nursing it must first be recognized that such an ethics exists within the influence of gender and politics as they relate to both men and women and

Condon, E. (1992, January/February). Nursing and the caring metaphor: Gender and political influences on an ethics of care. *Nursing Outlook*. Reprinted with permission of © *Nursing Outlook/* Mosby Yearbook. All rights reserved.

to ethics. Gender can be shown to impact upon an ethics of caring for nursing in a variety of ways. The first is the influence of social and biological con-structions of female gender. Since most nurses are women, this is significant. Riley (1988) tells us that the category *women* has undergone various con-structions and reconstructions reflecting a historical perspective on what it has meant to be a woman. She concludes that the category *women* is an unstable and vexed term for feminists who wish to create a political philosophy based on the experiences of women. She states, "modern feminism, which in its sociological aspects is landed with the identity of women as an achieved fact of history and epistemology, can only swing between asserting or refusing the completeness of this given identity" (p. 112).

THE HISTORICAL INFLUENCE OF GENDER

Historically, women, and their knowledge and point of view, have been either excluded entirely from conceptualizations of what it means to be human or have had their nature biologically, socially, or culturally defined in ways that have disturbed their identity. Women, it seems, have always been in transition toward, but never quite reaching, full human status or full partic-ipation in the given public, political, or spiritual domains. Women can never fully escape the influence of socially constructed gender that has variously overfeminized or underfeminized them, placing them in social roles that restrict their freedom of thought, will, and action (Riley, 1988; Rosenberg, 1982). The alleged inferiority of women is now seen as a historical and social construct of a masculine world view that has preempted full human partic-ipation of women in the world. Elshtain (1981), for example, utilizes the idea of the public and private domains as a prism through which to view women's oppression from ancient to modern times. In fact, the speech of women throughout history has been politically confined to the private world of the household. For Aristotle, "the household or private sphere represented a lesser good than the public sphere or polis. Exclusively private persons, not fully rational, limited in goodness, women lived out their lives in the realm of necessity, a life deemed inferior in its essence, intent, and purpose to political life but a functional prerequisite for the world of freedom" (p. 47).

In Elshtain's (1981) account, a public voice was the right and privilege of those who were declared to possess reason and goodness to its full extent. Politics, the sphere of action, the realm of the highest system of justice, was a space structured for an activity that served the end of the polis. By definition, public persons were responsible, rational, and free. They shared fully in private life and the life of the polis as its integral parts. Aristotle allowed no exceptions to the argument that the life of the whole was superior in nature, intent, and purpose to that of all "lesser" associations, including the family (pp. 46–47). Throughout Western, namely European, culture, influenced as it is by Aristotle, this privilege of a public voice is an ancient social and political precedent for the division of the public political sphere as dominated by men and the private sphere as inhabited by women.

Variations on this theme of inequality have played out for women throughout history. Whether they were defined as biologically defective and spiritually weak, or morally superior, women were confined to the private sphere with little public influence or political power or a voice in how public affairs should be conducted (Rosenberg, 1982). Confined to activities surrounding reproduction and care, women have continually found themselves under the authority of a patriarchal system of domination and control. Much of what women know about themselves and the world comes from knowledge constructed by men and does not fully account for their experience as female knowing subjects or for their ways of knowing (Belenky et al., 1986).

Feminists have approached the situation of women from various reflective standpoints, each having its own interpretation of the problems and corresponding solutions. Along this line, Benhabib (1987) has said that "although there is no agreement in the contemporary women's movement as to what the feminist vision of human liberation entails precisely, there is consensus around a minimal utopia of social life characterized by nurturant caring, expressive and non-repressive relationships between self and other, self and nature" (p. 5). Whether this will come about by overcoming the restrictions imposed by limited ways of conceptualizing gender, ethics, and politics, or by a revision of how gendered subjects ought to engage themselves ethically and politically, is as yet unknown. What is clear, however, is (1) that women's thinking and experience is challenging traditional ethical and political thinking, and (2) that as women contribute their knowledge to the world, change will be inevitable. One way in which nurses are likely to contribute to positive change in the way gender, ethics, and politics influence the public domain is through an exploration of the value and limitations of an ethics of caring for the profession. Since nurses participate in the public domain as members of a profession, they are in a position to contribute important insights about how an ethics of caring might positively influence the practice of nursing, ethics, and politics. Because nursing is practiced primarily by women, it is in the interest of nurses to explore modes of being ethical and political that reflect their lived experiences as women.

WOMEN AND CARING

According to Abel and Nelson (1990), caring is still a practice associated almost exclusively with women as a result of the sexual division of domestic labor in which women care not only for children but for disabled friends and relatives. Fisher and Tronto (1990) say that "caring is social because caring efforts speak ultimately to our survival as a species rather than isolated individuals. It is problematic because it involves social interactions that contain the potential for conflict and because it requires material resources that might be difficult or impossible to obtain" (p. 36). Because women have so much experience with caring, we tend to ignore it because we "know what it is" (p. 36). Women provide most of the caring activity in the home, community, and institutions designed to provide care. Because of the impersonal goals of bureaucratic systems, caregivers in institutions are frequently thwarted in their efforts to provide personalized holistic care, and their own status in the hierarchy intensifies the problem. Fisher and Tronto remark that "where responsibility is great but power is limited, women are expected to compensate for deficiencies in the caring process and the constraints of professionalization often limit caregivers' attention to a narrow sphere, so that it becomes difficult for them to approach a situation holistically" (p. 44).

Second wave feminist discourse has revealed three main images of caring. The selfish carer image arose as a response to the view that caring is a burden for women and that escape from the burden required that women put their own needs first. This view does explain how it accommodates care from others or whether or how we should ever care for anyone other than ourselves. The image of the androgynous carer arose from the hope that the inclusion of males in caring activities world increase its perceived value. Notwithstanding the positive value of that hope, it remains problematic. The entrenchment of caring in the sex/gender system and the sexual division of labor would require that radical changes here would require similar changes in the social construction of sexuality itself. It was also thought that the integration of males into caring work might create new patterns of male dominance in female helping professions. Here, the image of the visible carer developed from the argument that despite the disvaluing of women's caring due to the dominance of the male value system, caring should not be changed and women need not stop caring, but the worthiness of caring as an activity should be recognized, albeit via the enlistment of men. Recognition alone, however, whether via men or by the efforts of professional women carers, may not automatically assure an improved status for caring and may still result in avoiding or ignoring some aspects of caring linked to oppression

(Fisher & Tronto, 1990, 35–36). Finally, although caring has been shown to be integral to women's lives in the private and public sphere, it is noticeably absent from descriptions of "the good life" that provides the focus for Western philosophy, despite the fact that caring permeates our experience (p. 35). For feminists, however, there is a tendency to portray caring "as a positive dimension of our lives that has been socially devalued by a patriarchal or capitalist order" (p. 35). Given this background, let us examine what is meant by an ethics of caring and how it relates to nursing.

CURRENT MODELS OF INTERPERSONAL CARING

An ethics of care/caring has been described variously as a moral ideal of nursing (Watson, 1985) and a fundamental value of the nursing profession (Condon, 1988; Fry, 1989). Noddings's (1984) theory describes caring as an interpersonal process which forms the foundation of the ethical response in persons. She observes that caring has received attention only as an outcome of ethical behavior rather than as an underlying structure, which she believes motivates it. She states that the role of caring in the ethical response has been obscured by a prevailing masculine view of ethics and morality that emphasizes rules, logic, and justification, which, taken alone, are inadequate to concrete human situations.

For Noddings (1984), caring is a reciprocal but noncontractual process that does not involve any abstract notion of universal love, which she believes is unattainable and a distraction to caring. In contrast, Nodding emphasizes the particularity of the one cared for—there is no generalized other in a caring situation. With respect to roles, she believes that the role occupant is, first, one-caring and, second, enactor of specialized functions. This has important implications for nurses who may be socialized into expected role behaviors that consist of somewhat standardized responses to others. Noddings believes that since there can be no prior determination of what is fair or equitable in a particular situation, there can be no criterion to evaluate cases of caring. Such a criterion, in fact, would depend upon a number of conditions as viewed through the eyes of the person caring (one-caring) and the eyes of the cared for. In this context, *a priori* moral principles, rules, or criteria for justification are seen as irrelevant. Noddings also asserts that the demand for unquestioning obedience to the directives and rules of institutions contributes to the diminution of the ethical ideal of their members.

Gadow (1985) proposes that the moral quality of caring in nursing emerges from the idea of "commitment to a particular end . . . the protection and enhancement of human dignity" (p. 32). The caring relationship protects the patient from being reduced to the status of an object in the process of treatment of the patient's disease or resolution of the problem he or she is experiencing and, as such, protects his or her dignity. Truth-telling and touch are thought by Gadow to sustain the integrity and dignity of both nurse and client because both are subjectively engaged in the caring relationship. For Gadow, the particular versus the generalized other is the focus of the moral relationship.

Watson's (1985, 1988) "philosophy and theory of caring holds that caring is central to the practice of nursing and that it is transmitted by the culture of the profession as a unique way of coping with its environment" (1985, p. 8). Caring, Watson says, emerges from a humanistic-altruistic value system which "helps one to tolerate differences and to view others through their own perceptual systems rather than through one's own" (p. 11). Not only are individuals who are cared for expected to benefit from the interpersonal encounter with the caring nurse who relates to the client as "a valued person in and of him or herself to be cared for, respected, nurtured, understood and assisted" (1988, p. 14), the nurse also is expected to gain personally from the experience of caring. Such a basis for nursing (its philosophy or grounding ethic) when coupled with nursing as a human science is expected to contribute to the preservation of humanity. "Caring," according to Watson (1988), "is the moral ideal of nursing whereby the end is protection, enhancement, and preservation of human dignity" (p. 29). In this model, human caring involves both attitude and action directed toward a particular rather than a generalized other in a relationship with the nurse.

All such models of caring assume the participants in a caring process to be persons with histories, values, preferences, and differences, aspects which are expected to influence the process and outcomes of the caring encounter. The models emphasize the moral-relational rather than the labor aspect of caring and in this way expose an apparent feminine quality. The models reflect an expectation of mutuality and reciprocity in the caring relationship that would tend to limit, if not eliminate, exploitation or oppression of the carer at the individual if not at the bureaucratic level. It is noteworthy that all these theorists are women, two are nurses, and all are white, so their views may not reflect the diversity of perspectives that may exist about an ethics of caring as it is, or as it might be.

These models that are currently of interest to nurses seem also to reflect what Gilligan (1982, 1987) has characterized as an ethical orientation of care, of relationship and responsibility, which emerges from seeing issues within the context of relationships and the life situation of the particular other(s) involved rather than in the abstract context of the other viewed as some generalized entity to whom fixed rules and principles can be impartially applied in ethical situations. Although seeming to attribute a pattern of moral development for women that emphasizes responsibility and care as ethical responses, Gilligan does not rule out these kinds of responses for males also. Chodorow's (1978) theory of psychological development suggests also that the need for closeness, relatedness, and affection is a more likely outcome of female psychological development than of male development; thus, the tendency to see females rather than males as carers.

FEMINIST CRITIQUE OF A MODEL OF CARING

Although feminists have increasingly viewed the attribute of caring as a positive aspect of life, they have also critiqued it incisively. Criticisms of Noddings's ideas about caring center upon the potential for that construction of caring to be exploitive of the carer and the potential for that form of caring to be unavailable to, or exclusive of, men as a way of being ethical. Hoagland (1990) takes issue with Noddings's caring ethic on the basis of its reflecting a mothering model that, she says, puts carers at risk of exploitation by the ones they care for. She argues that Noddings's caring model is not reciprocal and that the caring goes only in one direction—from carer to one cared for with only minimal acknowledgement returning to the carer. This, she believes, reinforces the oppressive expectation that women should be selfless carers. Hoagland also objects to what she sees as the overemphasis of other-directedness of the model and its negative influence on the ethical identity of the carer whose only motivation for self-caring is that he or she can become a better one-caring. She believes that inherent in Noddings's model of feminine caring is a context of oppression. She sees this type of caring as "disconnected from political reality, material conditions, and social structure of the world" (p. 113).

Houston (1990) criticizes Noddings's concept of caring, citing, as one of its most oppressive features, a misplaced sense of responsibility in the one-caring for the one cared for, which could maintain the one-caring in possibly harmful relationships. Regardless of Noddings's claim that the form of caring that she envisions can be practiced by males, Houston is unconvinced that it would be due to the implacability of the ". . . gendered distribution of benefits and burdens of caring, and the fact that it is recognizably tied to the sexual division of labor which holds women responsible for nurturance and caretaking" (p. 118). For Houston (1989), this raises concerns related to the socialization of young girls into caring roles. Such socialization is potentially threatening to the ability of young girls to resist violence and exploitation at the hands of men.

Card (1990), by questioning Noddings's claim that caring can substitute for an ethics of principle, offers an additional critique of Noddings's model. Indeed, Card finds Noddings troublesome here because her model restricts ethical relationships to those that fall within the circle of relationships with people whom the carer actually knows, thereby implying that there is no ethical relationship to people whom the carer does not know. Card says that it is an ethics of principle, in this case justice, which governs an ethical relationship with many people (generalized others) we don't know and who have the potential to harm or be harmed by us. Card also indicates that ethical principles do not "necessarily abstract from special connections with particular others" but that an ethics of principle makes it possible to have cooperative relationships with more people than one could or should try to care for (p. 105). Card also offers this criticism: Noddings's (1990) model of caring does not seem to do anything to alleviate the serious problems of social injustice endured by people not known to the carer nor does it create opportunities for relationships with others who would not, due to past injustice, enter the world of the carer. As a result, Card sees the need to both supplement and limit care with justice.

In response to the criticism that the caring relationship she describes is unidirectional and therefore exploitive of the carer, Noddings (1990) states that much of the energy required to maintain caring relations comes from the cared for. The response of the cared for invests energy in the relationship, and while the contribution of the cared for may be different or unequal in kind, Noddings asserts that the carer receives something from the cared for which contributes to the carer's capacity to relate, to work, and to sustain caring. Noddings acknowledges that caring relationships can involve participants who may contribute to the relationship unequally, but this is not necessarily problematic because the roles of carer or cared for are not exclusively occupied by a given person. She states that in mature relationships, the roles of cared for and carer are occupied interchangeably by both persons in the relationship. She concedes, however, that in the case of necessarily unequal relations, different or unequal contributions to the relationship could be problematic. Noddings says that the claim that an individual does or tries to permanently occupy only the carer role is a martyrlike posture and a perversion of her concept of caring. She acknowledges that society could exploit carers in the same way that it exploits advocates of social welfare and opponents to capital punishment, but feels that this potential alone does not invalidate those theoretical stances. Noddings's model of caring emphasizes a moral education in which everyone must learn to care, thereby reducing the potential for exploitation.

To Houston's (1990) concern that a displaced sense of responsibility in the carer could maintain the carer in harmful relationships, Noddings (1990) responds that from a perspective of caring, we are all called upon to stop abuse, and that the acceptance of abusive behavior is a perversion of caring because it encourages uncaring behavior from the abuser. She agrees that it is necessary to withdraw from direct personal abuse to protect oneself and that both the abused and the abuser need to be surrounded by caring others who will not tolerate abusive behavior and who will support the abused. To Card's (1990) criticism that Noddings's concept of caring restricts caring relationships to people the carer actually knows, Noddings replies that where personal caring encounters are not possible, indirect forms of caring, through others, are possible. Using the example of a contribution of resources to needy persons at a distance who are not personally known to the carer, Noddings explains that the practical problems involved require that the carer communicate with trusted intermediaries who are able to personally complete the act of caring by assuring that the cared for receives the needed resources. She acknowledges Card's insight that a concept of justice is needed ". . . in critiquing institutional constraints that cannot be ignored or entirely eliminated" (Noddings, 1990, p. 122) but also states: ". . . I am not ready to say exactly how justice and care should be combined, and that discussion will have to be undertaken at a future time" (1990, p. 14). With respect to a justice concept, Noddings adds that much thought is required about what justice actually means to the persons involved; otherwise a culturally imposed notion of justice may result. Card, nonetheless, agrees that caring is more basic to human life than justice, which she says we can survive without but which she says makes life worth living.

An Ethics of Caring Within a Feminist Philosophy

The insistence upon the valuing of a particular individual in a specific context is integral to an ethics of caring grounded in interpersonal models of caring relationships. However, this presents difficulty for such an ethics because it departs from the traditional stance of the generalized other whose rights or good are generally under consideration within an ethics that has evolved from social and contract theory. Social contract theory reflects Kantian morality, which assumes taking a moral position in relation to a generalized other. Such an other stripped of context, individuality, history, needs, desires, and differences is incoherent—simply, no person exists in that state. By placing affective, desire, and other individual concerns into a category of personal versus moral decisions, these concerns are effectively excluded from the moral domain where public justice is decided. Benhabib (1987) offers further, if general, criticism of universalistic moral theories in the Western tradition from Hobbes to Rawls: The universality they defend is defined by the experiences of adult white males, which are then taken as representative of the experience of all persons. Within a traditional approach to ethics, women's experiences, in a manner parallel to the concrete particulars of a generalized *other*, are relegated to the private/personal domain, and the knowledge and context important to moral decision making for them is thus made private and excluded from the public domain of ethics knowledge.

According to Benhabib (1987), "women's moral judgment is more contextual, more immersed in the details of relationships and narratives. It shows a greater propensity to take the standpoint of the particular other; and women appear more adept at revealing feelings of empathy and sympathy required by this" (p. 78). Having inherited the dichotomy between autonomy and nurturance, independence and bonding, and the sphere of justice and the domestic-personal realm, contemporary universalistic moral theory (Benhabib, 1987) cannot accommodate the particular concrete other who is the subject of an ethics of caring.

Walker (1989) has proposed an alternative to the traditional universalistic understandings of morality that provides a supportive philosophical basis for an ethics of caring based on interpersonal rather than impersonal relationships. Fundamental to her ideas of an alternative epistemology for a feminist ethics is the rejection of a moral point of view that excludes from the moral context the individuality, relationships, history, needs, and context of the person in the situation. A feminist ethics, according to Walker (1989) would require "attention to particular persons as *a* if not *the* morally crucial epistemic mode" (p. 17). This calls for "distinctive sorts of understanding" (p. 17), which she says are characterized by Gilligan's description of contextual and narrative versus formal and abstract patterns of thinking where the latter "abstracts the moral problem from the interpersonal situation" while the former involves a "narrative of relationships that extends over time" (pp. 17–18). This very much describes the kinds of contextual knowledge that nurses often acquire in nursing situations.

By considering a particular person's "history, identity, and affective-emotional constitution, and the special context that is a relationship, with *its* history, identity, and affective definition, one comes to the narrative or location of a human being's feelings, psychological states, needs and understandings" (p. 18). Such understandings extend backward and forward in time beyond the present, so that to really understand a person's emotions, intentions, and other mental states, we need to observe them as they form patterns over time and tell a "kind of story" (p. 18). Without this kind of understanding, it will be difficult to know "how it is with others toward whom I will act, or what the meaning or consequences of any acts will be" (p. 18). Walker (1989) also stresses the importance of communication as a path to understanding that is often ignored in moral deliberations using the traditional model of the isolated, independent decision maker. She challenges the required stance of impersonality and distancing required of moral decision makers in the universalist moral tradition because it has "institutionalized indirect ways of relating as moral paradigms" and enforces "communicative and reflective strategies which are interpersonally evasive" (p. 22).

Walker (1989) cautions that the alternative epistemology she proposes for a feminist ethics should not result in a willingness to endorse particularism for personal or intimate relations and universalism for the large-scale or administrative context, or for dealing with unknown or little-known persons. She cautions also that the limitations of the universalist moral stance should be recognized when it is the only one that can be resorted to because in recognizing them we avoid "becoming comfortable with essentially distancing, depersonalizing, or paternalistic attitudes which may not really be the only resorts if roles and institutions can be shaped to embody expressive and communicative possibilities" (p. 23). Although such an ethics might not provide a complete answer to all problems, an ethics which espouses attention to the concrete and particular other in his or her situation is considered necessary in the public domain to transform institutions which are impersonal or depersonalizing.

It should be evident from the forgoing discussion that an ethics of caring would find a conceptually happy home in Walker's epistemology for a feminist ethics. This is an important point because actualization of an ethics of caring in nursing will depend on the mutual interaction of theories and philosophies compatible with an ethics of caring. An ethics of caring must be informed with relevant knowledge and must be provided with knowledge grounded in the actual caring work and experiences of nurses, bringing theory and practice together in action. Actualizing an ethics of caring that avoids features of oppression and exploitation will also depend on its emergence as a political philosophy capable of transforming institutions and the politics within which nursing is practiced, on removing bureaucratic barriers to caring practice, and on removing conditions that exploit nurses in the carer role.

CONCLUSION

Compatibility between an ethics for nursing and a feminist ethics holds certain promise for nursing and feminism. The formal adoption of an ethics of caring by nurses and feminists would strengthen support for it as a desirable social ethic as well. Although philosophies, theories, and models of caring relationships continually appear in the literature, there remain questions that will only be answered by research and theorizing sensitive to the diverse contexts and nuances of caring. Nor is caring all there might be to nursing, ethics, and politics although it seems to make sense as a foundational moral value in all of the contexts discussed thus far. There is risk that an ethics of caring that sees human beings as connected and responsible to each other will be viewed as "gendered" and thereby flawed, but there is no conclusive argument about caring that suggests that it could not or should not be practiced by everyone.

To the initial query of whether or not an ethics of caring is relevant for nursing, the answer is yes. Are gender and political influences upon caring likely to prove detrimental to a practice based on an ethics of caring? To this, the answer is yes and no. If caring is identified only with women and those care-taking activities that have been relegated to women, then the answer is yes. The answer is no if an ethics of caring can continue to be brought out of the private into the public domain as a part of the moral and not just the personal life. This can occur through a blend of philosophy and nursing, both of which are practiced in the public domain, informed by a feminist ethics of caring. Nurses, however, will also need to explore the ways in which an ideology of professionalism conflicts with an ethics of caring. To the question of whether an ethics of caring might prove liberating in both private and public life, the answer is that it has the potential to do so. A social ethics of caring is one of the ways to overcome the discrepancies between the demands of the private and public domains. If feminists adopt an ethics which supports a caring ethics, then the tendency to depoliticize caring through attaching its significance exclusively to the female and the nurse roles and denying its significance beyond that will be diminished. Will everyone agree that an ethics based on caring is a suitable foundation for nursing of practice? No, some will believe that caring will usurp the notion of nursing science as a basis for nursing. However, some might agree that an ethics of care should underlie a science of nursing.

Men have used metaphors historically to sustain a tension between what they do and create and other forces that, when juxtaposed in the metaphor, provide a vehicle which disconnects the self and others (Kittay, 1988). The metaphor of caring has evolved as a significant metaphor for nursing, one different from previous metaphors such as religious calling, duty in the battle against disease, and other seemingly masculine metaphors that evoke images of separateness or adversity. I believe that the caring metaphor is authentic in that it emerges from the direct experience of women in the world as mothers, nurturers of the young, old, and ill, and as nurses. The metaphor of caring in nursing functions not to disconnect but to connect the self and the other whose sameness and differentness the nurse is prepared to accept. It is in the practice of nursing that a space is created for this to happen. Despite a long exile in the private domain, an ethics of caring is becoming the subject of public discourse. Duty and calling, old masculine metaphors for nursing, have been uncritically accepted despite the fact that they do not reflect nurses' caring experiences. Caring, freely chosen, provides a new and infinitely more authentic metaphor grounded in the experience of women and capable of being practiced by anyone who chooses it as a social as well as a professional ethics.

DISCUSSION QUESTIONS

1. Patricia Gray's chapter addresses the work of Jean Watson, one of the theorists also cited by Condon. Gray questions Watson's lack of attention to gender. How could the feminist analyses discussed by Condon be incorporated into a revision of Watson's work to strengthen it against Gray's criticisms?

2. Condon presents the view that much public discourse, including discourse on ethics, has reflected masculine perspectives. Women's experiences and understandings are often excluded. Women of color have often said the same thing about feminism: it often reflects the understandings of only white, relatively privileged women. Condon also notes that the theorists she discusses are all white women. How might women of color or poor women respond to the models of caring and the ethics of caring discussed in this article? What might they be most skeptical about? What might they most want to emphasize and preserve?

3. At several points, Condon refers to the notion of "generalized others." This usually means that, for example, other people are ascribed certain rights and responsibilities regardless of any consideration of their particular situations, personalities, or living conditions. Thus

everyone may be granted a "right" of free speech regardless of their education background, gender, ethnicity, or moral standards. Moral reasoning, under this model of the "generalized other," then endeavors to apply these "general" rights to a specific situation (e.g., yelling "fire" in a crowded theater or speech which denigrates, insults, or threatens others). Thus one needs to decide which rights "apply" in certain situations.

The particularized model resists abstracting general rules from the contextual, embedded nature of human interaction. Thus a right to free speech is not particularly helpful unless one knows something about the nature of the people involved, their relationships, purposes, etc. Thus one's speech is only free to the extent it takes into account the accepting, supportive relationship envisioned by an ethics of caring.

Nurses have often criticized the "vested interest" of physicians: their self-interest (e.g., having an active, successful surgical practice) interferes with a full, nurturing consideration of the best interests of the patient. How would an ethics of caring as described by Condon deal with the self-interests of nurses (e.g., their desire to leave work precisely on time or their desire for higher wages or, for those in private practice, for more clients paying more money)? You might refer to the chapters by O'Neill or Turkoski for supplemental ideas.

REFERENCES

Abel, E., & Nelson, M. (1990). Circles of care: An introductory essay. In E. Abel & M. Nelson (Eds.), *Circles of care: Work and identity in women's lives.* New York: State University Press.

Belenky, M. F., Clinchy, B., Goldberger, H. R., & Tarule, J. M. (1986). *Women's ways of knowing.* New York: Basic Books.

Benhabib, S. (1987). The generalized and concrete other: The Kohlberg-Gilligan controversy and feminist theory. In S. Benhabib & D. Cornell (Eds.), *Feminism as critique.* Minneapolis: University of Minnesota Press.

Card, C. (1990). Caring and evil. *Hypatia,* 5(1):101–107.

Chodorow, N. (1978). *The reproduction of mothering: Psychoanalysis and the sociology of gender.* Berkeley: University of California Press.

Condon, E. (1988). Reflections on caring and the moral culture of nursing. *Virginia Nurse,* 56(4), 23–27.

Elshtain, J. (1981). *Public man, private woman*. Princeton, NJ: Princeton University Press.

Fisher, B., & Tronto, J. (1990). Toward a feminist theory of caring. In E. Abel & M. Nelson (Eds.), *Circles of care work and identity in women's lives*. New York: State University Press.

Fry, S. (1989). The role of caring in a theory of nursing ethics. *Hypatia*, 4(2), 88–103.

Gadow, S. (1985). Nurses and Patient: The caring relationship. In A. H. Bishop & J. R. Scudder (Eds.), *Caring, curing, coping* (pp. 31–43). Tuscaloosa: The University of Alabama Press.

Gilligan, C. (1982). *In a different voice*. Cambridge, MA: Harvard University Press.

Gilligan, C. (1987). Moral orientation and moral development. In E. F. Kittay & D. T. Meyers (Eds.), *Women and moral theory*. Totowa, NJ: Rowman and Littlefield.

Hoagland, S. (1990). Some concerns about Nel Noddings' caring. *Hypatia*, 5(1), 109–113.

Houston, B. (1989). Prologomena to future caring. In M. Brabeck (Ed.), *Who cares? Theory, research, and educational implications of an ethics of care*. New York: Praeger Publishers.

Houston, B. (1990). Caring and exploitation. *Hypatia*, 5(1), 115–119.

Kittay, E. (1988). Woman as metaphor. *Hypatia*, 3(2), 63–86.

Noddings, N. (1984). *Caring: A feminine approach to ethics and morals*. Berkeley: University of California Press.

Noddings, N. (1990). A response. *Hypatia*, 5(1), 111–126.

Riley, D. (1988). *Am I that name? Feminism and the category of "women" in history*. Minneapolis: University of Minnesota Press.

Rosenberg, R. (1982). *Beyond separate spheres*. New Haven, CT: Yale University Press.

Walker, M. (1989). Moral understandings: Alternative "epistemology" for a feminist ethics. *Hypatia*, 4(2), 15–28.

Watson, J. (1985). *Nursing the philosophy and science of caring*. Boulder: Colorado Associated University Press.

Watson, J. (1988). *Human science and human care*. Norwalk, CT: Appleton Century-Crofts.

6

A Feminist Critique of Jean Watson's Theory of Caring

D. Patricia Gray

MY CONTEXT

During the past six years, I have been studying Jean Watson's work and the concept of caring. I have had an opportunity to spend time with Jean, and I have been profoundly influenced by her work on the concept of caring in nursing. Shortly after beginning my study of caring, I began to study feminist philosophy with Kay Hagan (1989, 1991). I have been influenced by the works of feminists Marilyn Frye (1983), Jeffner Allen (1990), bell hooks (1987, 1990), Patti Lather (1991), Sonya Johnson (1987), Mary Daly (1978, 1984), and many others. My life has been enriched by the day-to-day examples of living as a feminist provided to me by Joanne DeMark. I consider myself a radical feminist with sensitivity to the postmodern criticisms of the radical perspective. In addition, during the past three years, I have explored the works of Alice Miller (1983, 1984) whose ideas about the development of family dynamics have contributed to my understanding of why I am concerned about caring. Bradshaw's (1988) practical application of Miller's work has been helpful to me in exploring how my upbringing in a dysfunctional family affected me and has influenced my professional career and personal life. I have examined the literature on co-dependency during the past two years, and I maintain a concern regarding the tensions between caring and co-dependency.

I also find myself drawn to three principles suggested by Joyce Trebilcot in her essay, "Dyke Methods" (Trebilcot, 1990). These principles reflect values I hold today as I share my ideas with you:

- I speak only for myself;
- I do not try to get other women to accept my beliefs in place of their own.
- There is no given (that is, every patriarchal assumption, every axiom of received reality, is ultimately to be questioned for the purpose of deciding whether to accept it as it is, change it or reject it entirely; all the alleged immutables of nature, of the human condition, of ultimate reality, must be identified and evaluated (p. 22).

THE CRITIQUE

Why a critique of Watson's theory of caring? I believe that caring is a potentially liberating concept, and I am passionately concerned about how the concept is developed so that it is truly emancipatory, rather than a concept that reinforces aspects of dominant culture, especially power-over relations and misogyny. Studying feminism, I've come to understand the subleties of dominant culture and the power of dominant culture to prescribe what is "good" for people. Growing up in and participating in dominant culture, I have also grown more and more aware of how many of the values and methods of dominant culture I've accepted as my own. I am especially concerned that in taking on some, if not all, of the patriarchal representations of caring that I am accepting perspectives that tend to deny or obscure some aspects of caring while highlighting others. Specifically, I am concerned that my training in dominant culture makes it difficult for me to: (1) identify, in particular, what is obscured and (2) remember that that which is highlighted is highlighted to reinforce values and perspectives of dominant culture. This chapter, then, represents part of the journey of my uncovering what is obscured and my reexamining what is emphasized by dominant culture. In effect, I am claiming *my* power to determine what is "good" for me.

Therefore, while caring is a very appealing concept to me, I want to be clear about the ways in which I undertake to practice caring and to be in the world in caring ways. I also want to understand the ways in which patriarchal culture has influenced my experiences of caring and possibly limited my understanding of the potential of caring. Within this context, what does Jean Watson have to say to me about caring?

Milton Mayeroff (1971) makes the observation that we sometimes speak as if caring did not require knowledge; however, he notes that in order to care, we must know many things (p. 13). Jean Watson's work on caring has focused awareness on caring and has made explicit the knowledge required to engage in caring. This is a significant contribution to the discipline and profession of nursing. Her work on caring has and will continue to shape conversations we have with each other about nursing and its nature.

One aspect of this conversation is a process of reflexive and critical questioning. Although two main questions regarding Watson's theory appear equally, I am also aware of a general concern about theory in general. I address this general question first.

It is my uncomfortable suspicion that theory, or perhaps the ways in which we use theory, tends to foster the replication of dominant culture, especially relationships of domination and subordination. Maria Lugones and Elizabeth Spellman (1990) address this issue in their wonderful essay, "Have we got a theory for you," in which they ask probing questions about theory itself:

> What are the things we need to know about others, and about ourselves in order to speak intelligently, sensitively, and helpfully about their lives? When we speak, write, and publish our theories, to whom do we think we are accountable? Are the concerns we have in being accountable to "the profession" at odds with the concerns we have in being accountable to those about whom we theorize? Do commitments to "the profession," method, getting something published, getting tenure, lead us to talk and act in ways at odds with what we ourselves (let alone others) would regard as ordinary, decent behavior? To what extent do we presuppose that really understanding another person or culture requires our behaving in ways that are disrespectful, even violent? Why and how do we think theorizing about others provides understanding of them? Is there any sense in which theorizing about others is a short-cut to understanding them? (p. 30)

Lugones and Spelman, recognizing the limitations of the language of theory, call for the meaningful involvement of diverse voices in its creation. They suggest that such involvement requires openness, sensitivity, concentration, self-questioning, circumspection, and a giving up of the assumed authority of knowledge.

Related concerns are raised by bell hooks (1989) in her book *Talking Back*. She discusses some of the problems she experiences with theory, namely that it is inaccessible and is often created by white, middle-class academics who lack an understanding of the perspectives of women of color. As she says, "Increasingly, one type of theory is seen as valuable—that which is Euro-centric, linguistically convoluted and rooted in Western white male sexist and racially biased philosophical frameworks" (p. 36). Elitism and racial blindness or invisibility tend to maintain current power-over dynamics. Hooks suggests the creation of theory that is accessible and that involves all kinds of women, many modes of dissemination, many kinds of discourse, and many divergent points of view.

The words of these women support me in beginning to question. I look at the ways in which language is used in theory and for the voices reflected in the theory. I begin to assess my participation in theorizing, and I examine how my views on theory influence my behavior and dialogue with others. I ask, as I theorize, as I use theory, how do I participate in the "authority of knowledge"? What are the things I need to know about myself as a nurse, theorist, and researcher?

How do I use theory? I notice that I have the capacity to question, and I notice a coexisting conditioned response to authority. Theory and theo-retical undertakings seem intellectually imposing. *Theory, science, power, authority*—these words all seem related. I notice my conditioned response to someone with perceived power—a dean of a school of nursing, someone with a PhD, someone whose work has been published, an "expert" in the field of caring. I tend to discount my questions, rationalize about why I shouldn't have these (or any) questions. I recognize my well-developed response as a received knower, and I notice that I constrain my thinking about caring to the frame of reference outlined in "the" theory. I notice that I read Jean Watson's work from that perspective of "oh how delightful—now someone is going to tell me about caring and what it is about." My working assumption seems to be that her experience is more valuable than mine, that her way of illuminating the world of caring is more significant, because she is more knowledgeable than I am, because she has published, because she is in some way more than I am. Let me be clear here—none of this has anything to do with Jean Watson, her theory, or her intent in publishing her work—it is simply a reflection of one way I can choose to be with it—and perhaps this is not an uncommon choice. Based on my long conditioning as a received knower, as described by Belenky (1985), how else might I expect myself to react to a theory? As a received knower, I viewed theory as an absolute statement of scientific authority. Yet I return to my observation that I do question in spite of my conditioning as a received knower, and I return again and again to the questions. I am also aware that some part of my experience must support me in the process of exploration, of questioning.

Watson begins her second book, *Nursing: Human Science and Human Care* (1985) with a discussion of theory, theory development, and the evolution of science in nursing. She advocates a very liberal view of theory, which she defines as "an imaginative grouping of knowledge, ideas and experience that are represented symbolically and seek to illuminate a given phenomenon" (p. 1). I question: Whose imagination? Whose ideas and experience? Knowledge created by whom? What are the symbolic representations? By whom are they created? Who uses which symbols in what ways? Illumination— who creates the light and then directs its beam? Who chooses what is illuminated?

In the scientific realm, theory has another purpose not addressed by Watson—to predict and control. Although I appreciate that Watson is suggesting other uses for theory, theory itself continues to be considered prescriptive by many. Given that theory is a value-laden enterprise, the purpose of prediction and control becomes a political enterprise—and one that I take very seriously. As a woman who has been construed, predicted, and controlled by dominant culture, I am skeptical of efforts related to perpetuating this cycle in my life. My goal is to claim my experience as valid for myself, to take charge of my own destiny by being clear about the reality I am creating for myself through my beliefs and perceptions. Within this context, what role does theory play? Although my experience is that theory tends to obscure difference and diversity and to constrain dialogue, is this how I use theory rather than something inherent about the nature of theory?

Perhaps prematurely, I leave this reflection on theory, recognizing that I am a part of the system that I am questioning; to some extent, this limits the questions I consider and determines the language I use. I am aware that I may be using the tools of that which I critique in this process of questioning; I may be less aware of all the ways in which I use those tools.

I move to consider aspects of Jean Watson's theoretical formulations about caring. I have two specific concerns: (1) the theory of caring that Watson articulates is ungendered, and (2) Watson's theory is focused on the transpersonal, spiritual dimensions of relationship.

My first concern is related to the ungenderedness of Jean Watson's theory of caring. The absence of gender as related to the concept of caring implies that gender is unrelated or irrelevant to the concept of caring. Since gender is not mentioned in the development of this theoretical formulation, opportunities may be minimized for dialogue concerning the issue of gender in relationship to caring. I wonder, is "caring" a universal phenomenon that transcends the people doing it? Do men and women "do" caring differently? How do female nurses experience caring, and how does their experience as women influence their caregiving for males and females, adults and children?

A similar question could be asked for male nurses. Are caring activities received differently by clients, depending on the gender of the caregiver and the gender of the client (Kuharcik, 1987)? How does Watson's experience as a woman contribute to how she understands caring in contrast to, for example, Mayeroff's understanding of caring?

Watson raises important issues in her statement of assumptions. She states that "we have to treat ourselves with gentleness and dignity before we can respect and care for others with gentleness and dignity" (p. 33). If gender were addressed in this theory of caring, questions might be raised such as: "Is learning to treat ourselves with gentleness and dignity a different process for men and women, for whites and people of color, for members of other dominant groups and people of other subordinate groups?" Learning to shed my internalized sexism, for example, has been an incredibly powerful yet time- and energy-consuming process for me. It was a process foundational to my ability to treat myself with gentleness and dignity. Watson further notes in her assumptions that human care, at the individual and group level, has received less and less emphasis in the health care delivery system and that caring values of nurses and nursing have been submerged. I wonder if these statements of value are related to the fact that over 95 percent of nurses in the United States are women, that caring is considered women's work, and that women's work remains greatly undervalued? Certainly, an inclusion of gender in Watson's theory would provide opportunities to explore these issues in greater depth and lead to more meaningful understandings of the gender-relatedness of caring. Finally, I have serious concern, given the preferential valuing of maleness in our culture, that an ungendered theory assumes maleness as the norm, thus perpetuating many values of dominant culture. One way in which a dominant culture value may be replicated is in the language of the theory, which, again, tends to be white, Eurocentric, and based on male-dominated philosophical frameworks.

A second concern here regards Jean Watson's focus on the transpersonal, spiritual dimensions of relationship. "The art of transpersonal caring allows humanity to move towards greater harmony, spiritual evolution and perfection" (p. 74). I found this aspect of Watson's theory very compelling as I first read her work. The transpersonal, spiritual aspects of relationship have been very important to me. However, Watson's focus on the transpersonal and spiritual has had the effect of shifting my attention away from my physical existence and from the physical aspects of relating to and caring for others. This shift is congruent with a social valuing of the spiritual as something "light," "clean," and "higher" and a devaluing of the physical as "dirty" and "lower." I have become increasingly aware that the body has been described and viewed as dirty, as a source of sin, for example, particularly with regards to relating to others (Dworkin, 1976). A transcendental focus shifts me away from these dirty, "distasteful" aspects of my existence, and I am less inclined to explore the physical aspects of caring. Yet I increasingly recognize my physical body as my personal historian—the memory of every event in my life, every feeling, stored somewhere in my physical body. I need access to that part of myself if I am to *engage in caring* and become fully authentic— to claim fully who I am—since that includes not only what I want to become but what I have been and experienced. A focus away from my physical self is an easier path for me, because being a woman in the world has been a relatively painful experience for me. Part of me welcomes an opportunity to avoid focusing on my physical body. And now I realize that to take that approach is to deny part of myself. This is not to say that Watson does not acknowledge the physical body—certainly in her carative factors, the physical body is addressed. Yet the physical body and its place in relationship, an acknowledgement of the labor it provides, for example, is not sufficiently addressed. Other questions remain for me as well: In what ways can physical relationships between people be caring? In what important ways are nurses' relationships with patients physical (not sexual) relationships?

Watson's ideas about the transpersonal aspects of caring have been heavily influenced by Eastern spiritual philosophy. My spiritual practices have also been influenced by these same philosophies. However, I share Mary Daly's (1985) concern that major religious traditions do not acknowledge or affirm women's experiences, but rather work to use women's energies to achieve their own goals. Additionally, some aspects of Eastern philosophy are deeply troubling to me—for example, the Hindu belief that heterosexuality is necessary for spiritual evolution to one's highest potential. While Watson's theory does not address issues of heterosexism, the absence of such a discussion might lend implicit support to this aspect of the Eastern spiritual perspective.

These concerns reflect a growing distrust I am noticing regarding the partial adaptation of a theory or perspective. Andrea Nye (1988) has described a metaphor for creating a new tapestry using the threads from other philosophies, other tapestries. She suggests that it is extremely difficult to extract a single thread from another tapestry, in that it might continue to be attached to its original source. The image that comes to my mind is a tapestry woven from threads that carry major unintended pieces of other tapestries—not a particularly aesthetic image. What are the consequence of creating our caring tapestry in this way? Are there other ways to create a tapestry of caring? (As an aside, Nye suggests that we can learn many things as we unravel male-dominated traditions. Do I want to spend my time unraveling these traditions, or are there other ways to spend my time?)

As I reflect on the use of Eastern traditions, I also ask whether there is evidence to support the implication that Eastern approaches lead one to a more caring view of oneself or the world. Have Eastern ways of relating to each other resulted in more caring interactions, more caring relationships? These are questions which are still with me.

NEW DIRECTIONS

Based on my initial concern about theory, my present goal is to develop for myself a clear understanding of how I am in the world and how my being can be in interaction with others in ways that are affirming and empowering and, thus, caring. This understanding is grounded in experiencing myself as a physical being engaged in physical labor, the expenditure of energy on my behalf and the behalf of others. As a woman, I further recognize myself as a human being whose physical body is denied and forbidden to me in ways both subtle and obvious. I therefore claim the forbidden for myself.

I believe that the mechanics of my way of being will not necessarily be helpful to others. I have chosen certain goals for myself that may be relevant to others, if others choose to adopt these goals for themselves. These include finding a voice, claiming my power, and being fully authentic. It may be that agreeing on these goals creates a community of nursing that is caring. The form of that caring would be in process, individual and evolving. Do we need theory to help us work that out?

RECENT REFLECTIONS

I presented this work at two conferences during 1989 and 1990. At both conferences, concern was expressed that I had criticized Jean Watson's theory of caring. Because caring is an important and meaningful concept to me, my critique is offered in the spirit of developing our scholarly dialogue about caring to expand its emancipatory potential. As Peggy Chinn noted at the 1991 Summer Institute on Human Caring, caring is not about "making nice." It is about taking the time and energy to share concerns when those concerns are present.

Since I initially presented this paper, I have continued to reflect upon ways in which my thinking about caring is enhanced and constrained by "theories" *of* or *about* caring. I notice that students talk about Watson's theory of caring as if it is something static, written in concrete. I hear them discuss ways in which their research or their experience "fits" the theory. I am disturbed that I do not hear conversations about their theories of caring. I wonder when we will remember that while we can appreciate the beauty of the theory that Watson has created, we also need to spend time on creating, developing, and explicating our own perspectives on caring. I am convinced that these personal explorations of caring are as important as Watson's perspectives on caring, and I am concerned that theory in general continues to limit our imagination.

I also continue my struggle with theory and its usefulness to me. My current perspective is very personal. In her book *Feminist Theory and the Philosophies of Man*, Andrea Nye (1988) says, "Theory has its origins in neither nature nor logic, but in the struggle to make sense of human action" (p. 230). Over the past three years, I have struggled to make sense of my growing-up years, of the pain I experienced as a child. I have come to understand that in my desire to survive my childhood emotional, physical, and sexual abuse, I moved away from the physical and emotional experiences of my life and lived in a castle of abstractions that I created and expanded as I needed—a castle with very thick walls that protected me from pain and isolated me from my experiences. I created my own personal ivory tower of theory to help me make sense of human action around me. Nye asserts that theory is a linguistic structure in which men escape their physicality and their emotional needs (p. 230). I discovered that I used the same survival strategy.

Now, as a researcher, when I contemplate the notion of the "lived world" or the "lived experience," I realize that I don't know what that means and I have no idea about how to access it for myself. Having a direct experience, not mediated by or through theory, is something difficult for me to imagine. How do people do it? Do people do it?

I assume at this time that my lived experience is one lived in and through theory—through the thick castle walls of abstraction. This realization came to me at a qualitative research conference as I listened to women present their research findings without benefit of theoretical underpinnings that, in my estimation, would have greatly improved or enhanced their analyses. Yet these researchers were able to do something incredibly important, especially to a qualitative researcher. They were able to have and report their direct experiences, and I felt intense sadness to realize the extent to which I was separated from my experience by my theorizing.

Alice Miller describes the effects of childhood experiences on later life choices and experiences. Her analysis of Nietzsche (Miller, 1990) helped me see that my childhood probably has had an influence on my academic undertakings in ways that I am just coming to understand. I understand that I continue to use a survival strategy of theorizing and intellectualizing that I developed at a very young age. I recognize that I have valued theory to help protect me from the "real" world. I have spent most of my intellectual life learning how to use language in scholarly ways designed to impress others and to distract and distance me from the pain of my everyday lived world. My real world is a world of words, ideas, abstractions. I rationalize and intellectualize as a primary mode of being. I struggle against the split between the intellectual and the experiential, and I discover that split within myself. I asked in the conclusion of my paper, do we need theory? My answer at this point is that I don't have any idea how to approach the world except through the lens of theory, through the distancing language of theoretical abstraction. My current focus is on embracing my use of theory as a strength and on nurturing and supporting my explorations into the world of things and people and relationships—another "real" world.

I end with sharing a piece that I wrote several years ago and read last year at the Critical and Feminist Perspectives in Nursing Conference. This piece has assumed new meaning for me over the past year.

New Faces in the Crowd

Faces of academic elitism
> *Research, theory, knowledge, science,*
> *evaluation, funding, rank.*
> *All embracing traditional structures of domination*
> *(they don't call it the Ivory Tower for nothin').*
And another one joins the crowd
> *Feminist theory*
> *A sterile, linguistically convoluted body*
> *formed using western white male models,*
> *speaking an alienating language of rationality.*
> *Breasts that give nourishment to the intellectual elite*
> *a barren womb struggling to give birth to emancipation.*
Yet another version of authoritarian discourse
> *evolving from our participation*
> *within institutions selling unconsciousness*
> *and self-hatred as truth.*
> *Institutions espousing values,*
> *modes of thought and ways of being*
> *that entice us into forgetting who we are,*
> *what we know, how we know it.*

And still, we remember.
  In spite of the form
  in spite of the context
  we question, we heal ourselves.
  With theory, through theory,
  in spite of theory—we remember.
And in the remembering, we claim
  our power to create in our own image,
  our voice to speak our own language.
  We invoke a merging of theory
  and experience and in so doing,
  we open doors and minds and vistas
  to new modes of being.
The face of feminist theory is changing.
  And so am I.

DISCUSSION QUESTIONS

This paper raises at least three questions: (1) a general questioning of theory and its uses; (2) questions regarding caring as a gendered activity; and (3) questions about "weaving" patriarchal ideas and practices into nursing.

1. Why has theory become problematic for Gray? What are the problems created by theorizing? What enabling functions does theory provide?

2. How does the consideration of gender alter a discourse about caring? When gender is made explicit in a discourse of care, what effect does this have on previous notions about "humanistic caring?"

3. As Gray explores the question of "weaving" patriarchal ideas and practices (e.g., transcendence) into nursing, she is ambivalent. Do you share this ambivalence? If so, why?

4. Like other papers in this collection, Gray resists the constructions of dominant culture in nursing. What does she mean by acknowledging that postmodern feminists have challenged her thinking? Can she claim a "woman-centered" space as a location for nursing? Why/not? How is this problem similar to questions raised by Thompson, Skillings, Turkoski, and Allman?

REFERENCES

Allen, J. (Ed.). (1990). *Lesbian philosophies and cultures.* New York: SUNY Press.

Belenky, M., et al. (1985). *Women's ways of knowing.* New York: Basic Books.

Bradshaw, J. (1988). *Bradshaw on the family.* Deerfield Beach, FL: Health Communications.

Daly, M. (1978). *Gyn-ecology: The metaethics of radical feminism.* Boston: Beacon Press.

Daly, M. (1984). *Pure lust: Elemental feminist philosophy.* Boston: Beacon Press.

Daly, M. (1985). *The Church and the second sex.* Boston: Beacon Press.

Dworkin, A. (1976). *Women hating: A radical look at sexuality.* New York: Dutton.

Frye, M. (1983). *The politics of reality.* Freedom, CA: The Crossing Press.

Hagan, K. (1989). *Internal affairs.* San Francisco: Harper and Row.

Hagan, K. (1991). *Prayers to the moon.* San Francisco: Harper and Row.

hooks, b. (1987). *From margin to center.* Boston: South End Press.

hooks, b. (1989). *Talking back.* Boston: South End Press.

hooks, b. (1990). *Yearning: Race, gender and cultural politics.* Boston: South End Press.

Johnson, S. (1987). *Going out of our minds: The metaphysics of liberation.* Freedom, CA: The Crossing Press.

Kuharcik, K. (1987). *Patients' experiences of being cared-for in the coronary care unit.* Unpublished master's thesis, Georgia State University, Atlanta, GA.

Lather, P. (1991). *Getting smart.* New York: Routledge.

Lugones, M., and Spelman, E. (1990). Have we got a theory for you. In al-Hibri, A. (Ed.), *Hypatia reborn.* Bloomington: Indiana University Press.

Mayeroff, M. (1971). *On caring.* New York: Harper and Row.

Miller, A. (1983). *For your own good.* New York: Farrar, Straus, Giroux.

Miller, A. (1984). *Thou shalt not be aware.* New York: Farrar, Straus, Giroux.

Miller, A. (1990). *The untouched key.* New York: Farrar, Straus, Giroux.

Nye, Andrea (1988). *Feminist theory and the philosophies of man.* London: Croom Helm.

Trebilcot, J. (1990). Dyke methods. In Allen, J. (Ed.), *Lesbian philosophies and cultures.* New York: SUNY Press.

Watson, J. (1985). *Nursing: Human science and human care.* Norwalk, CT: Appleton Century Crofts.

7

Reproductive Technology and Court Ordered Obstetrical Interventions: The Need for a Feminist Voice in Nursing

Elizabeth I. Hagell

Procreation has always been a social event and every society has legal, medical or ethical rules about birthing and childbirth. Unfortunately, the childbearers (women) have usually not been the rule makers, and too often women's health and interests have been controlled by or subordinated to the concerns of dominant males. (Canadian Research Institute for the Advancement of Women [CRIAW] 1989, p. 2)

Hagell, E. I. (1991). Reproductive technology and court ordered obstetrical interventions: The need for a feminist voice in nursing. *Health Care for Women International*. Reprinted with permission. ©Health Care for Women International. All rights reserved.

INTRODUCTION

CRIAW has identified clearly the very broad issues surrounding reproduction. Nurses are closely connected to these concerns as practitioners, as
women, and as promoters of health. Researchers in nursing have been seemingly reluctant to address the issues regarding nursing's role and practice in
relation to reproductive health care. As the development and increasing use
of reproductive technologies continues, as court ordered obstetrical interventions occur, and as calls for "fetal abuse" laws and more restrictive abortion
legislation continue, questions regarding nursing's role become increasingly
important.

In this paper I will identify issues surrounding reproductive technologies,
court ordered obstetrical interventions, other developments in the area of
reproductive health care, and examine how the nursing literature has dealt
with these issues. Mine is an attempt to encourage nurses to examine and
discuss these developments from a critical woman-centered approach that
places women at the center of any discussion and that attempts to understand
these measures in a social and historical context, in other words, a feminist
perspective.

I reviewed published nursing journal literature for the five-year period from
1985 to 1990 after decisions related to definitions and criteria were established. The search included the *Cumulative Index to Nursing and Allied Health
Literature* as well as a computerized literature search conducted by the Organization for Obstetric, Gynecologic and Neonatal Nurses Association
(NAACOG). I reviewed literature using these subject headings: fertilization,
artificial; insemination, artificial; reproduction; fetal versus maternal rights;
and trends in American reproductive technologies. All articles were examined
and grouped together based on the concerns identified and approach or
subjects studied.

To date, most researchers in nursing who have examined reproductive
technologies, for example, have done so from a psychological or "coping"
perspective of the couple (Milne, 1987). Others have examined the technical
advances (Olshansky, 1988; Pace-Owens, 1985) and the ethical problems
created by the use of reproductive technologies (Francis & Nosek, 1988;
Poteet & Lamar, 1986).

The majority of these researchers view reproductive technologies as either
acceptable technologies or as technologies that may create ethical dilemmas
that must be legislated or controlled. Very few researchers in nursing have
identified concerns regarding the recent developments in reproductive technologies from a feminist perspective. Even fewer researchers in nursing have

addressed the question of court ordered obstetrical interventions (Kroll, 1987; Twomey, 1989).

The lack of a feminist or critical, woman-centered approach for nurses and nursing has broad and far-reaching implications. If nurses do not understand and speak about these issues, they may find themselves on the outside of important debates about society and health. Indeed, in almost all mainstream and feminist literature related to reproductive technologies and court ordered obstetrical interventions nurses are invisible. One would assume from reading the material that nurses were not involved. Only one researcher (Williams, 1989) examines the role of nurses in supporting and implementing these measures. The lack of a strong woman-centered voice in nursing has serious consequences as nurses continue to strive for increased autonomy and respect. Nurses who are involved directly in reproductive health care, as well as nurses generally, must become more critical of these developments. It is crucial that questions be asked about both the underlying assumptions of these measures and about the implications of these assumptions for the women involved as patients and nurses. Otherwise, nurses may unwittingly support technologies and other measures which harm women and nursing itself.

Important here is an examination of the major issues identified in the mainstream and feminist literature, as well as in nursing literature, in relation to reproductive technologies to determine, in this context, current approaches to research. I will also address the particular issues involved in court ordered obstetrical interventions. Although these may seem like rather diverse topics, there are underlying themes and assumptions that are common to their development. Finally, I will offer the beginnings of an analysis, using feminist theory, that will help nurses to understand more clearly why they must question their role in the implementation and support of noted developments and their consequences in reproductive technology.

REPRODUCTIVE TECHNOLOGIES

It has been over a decade since Louise Brown, the world's first "test-tube" baby was born in 1978. She was conceived using a procedure called in vitro fertilization (IVF). Since that time, there have been other developments in reproductive technologies including nonsurgical embryo transfer procedures, sex selection, and fetal therapy. IVF clinics now exist worldwide, from Canada and the United States to Brazil and South Africa. In 1987, there were 12 clinics in Canada and 150 clinics in the United States. According to Pappert (1988), almost 3,500 women have tried IVF.

Along with these technological developments, there has been a great deal written about reproductive technology in the mainstream literature of philosophy, sociology, and psychology as well as in the more specialized fields of medicine and jurisprudence that questions its benefits and its implementation. In all this diverse material, commonly held, general concerns surface repeatedly. As summarized by Koch & Morgall (1987), Moss (1988), and Williams (1986), they include ethical and legal considerations, questions about the social implications of such technologies, concerns about changing social roles, and social structure and economic issues. A brief examination of each of these issues may be useful in clarifying these concerns.

Numerous questions regarding ethical and legal issues are raised by reproductive technologies. Questions surrounding the legal status of the fetus, ownership and control of embryos, and the use of embryos for research are but a few that the courts have already had to deal with. In response to these questions, commissions of inquiry have been formed and reports have been issued by various legal groups. For example, in Canada, the Ontario Law Reform Commission (1985) produced a lengthy document, *Report on Human Artificial Reproduction and Related Matters*. In Great Britain, *The Warnock Report* (in Spallone, 1986) attempted to address these issues. The Department of the Interior in Denmark (1984), as well as the state government in Queensland, Australia (1984), also produced reports on reproductive technologies. Although the recommendations found in these reports differ somewhat in their approach to controlling and legislating reproductive technologies, one consistent aspect is the lack of a perspective which recognizes the special nature of human reproduction and its significance for women. Indeed, these reports accept many assumptions about women and women's roles and view reproductive matters as any contractual or property issue (Williams, 1986; Spallone, 1990).

Questions about the social implications of reproductive technologies center about the question of gene manipulation and eugenics. Some authors relate current work in reproductive technology to the eugenics movement (Hubbard, 1987; Singer & Wells, 1984). Although these concerns are not without merit, their social implications for women have not been addressed or even acknowledged.

Another identified area of concern relates to questions of social roles and control of reproductive technologies. For example, the selection process for any of the available technologies, from sperm donation to in vitro fertilization, seems to favor white, middle-class individuals. What are the criteria for selection, and how were they developed? In addition, questions related to the definition of parenthood become very obscure and ill-defined here. At this point in time, a child could potentially have a biological mother, a biological father, a birth mother, a social mother, and a social father all of whom are different people.

Another concern related to reproductive technologies involves questions of cost. Not only are obvious questions of concern, such as how much people pay for in vitro fertilization (for example, some estimates are as high as three to fiye thousand dollars per attempt), but also of concern are questions about whether reproductive technologies treat children, sperm, eggs, and embryos as commodities.

It quickly becomes clear that many vital questions about reproductive technologies and their implications for women remain to be answered. That mainstream discussions of reproductive technologies consistently avoid their effect on women, however, is striking. As Warren (1988) notes, "thus far little of the public debate about the ethics of IVF and other reproductive technologies has focused upon the possible negative effects of these technologies on women" (p. 37).

In response, feminist writers and researchers are turning their attention to new developments in reproductive technologies. However, it is important to understand that the feminist position on reproductive technologies has been neither uniform nor consistant over time. Shulasmith Firestone (1979), for one, took the radical stance of believing that only the reproduction of children outside the womb would be necessary for the liberation of women. More recently, as discussed by O'Brien (1981), feminist theorists have taken a contrary tack, turning their attention to childbearing and reproduction and attempting to understand how the capacity to bear children shapes women's consciousness and their lives. When examined in this light, of course, the impact of reproductive technologies takes on greater meaning. Nonetheless, while feminists express various, and sometimes conflictive, views on the future role of reproductive technologies, they also agree there are many questions that remain to be answered.

A document by CRIAW (1990) notes, "Because the lives of women are so personally affected by the reproductive technologies their voices must direct the discussion concerning public. policy and legislation. A woman-centred perspective on human reproduction explores and gives voice to women's experiences" (p. 4). As noted earlier, CRIAW and others have criticized previous reports for not having a women-centered approach, for taking the male perspective as the norm, and for remaining unaware of the different ways in which women may experience the world. In regard to the Warnock report, for example, CRIAW points out that while it does "address the problems that IVF may hold for people with certain religious beliefs, for those that believe in the sanctity of the embryo, and for those concerned about the cost of the program," it "does not address the problems that IVF poses for the woman whose health is at risk for the sake of a technology with a 80–100 percent failure rate."

Such a perspective, which could be called nonfeminist, also tends to dismiss the reality of sexual inequality in our society, thereby reinforcing women's subordination. Spallone (1987), for exammple, calls the approach of these reports "embryo-centred and knowledge-centred not woman-centred" (p. 168).

Other authors, such as Koch and Morgall (1987), Moss (1988), and Warren (1988) have summarized significant feminist concerns regarding reproductive technologies as follows:

1. The further medicalization of the female body and normal biological processes. The history of male intervention in women's reproductive processes has not been an illustrious one. Many feminist writers (e.g., Ehrenreich & English, 1979; Oakley, 1986; Rich, 1986) have documented the problems of the male medical model.

2. The ongoing male domination of the health care system and of the reproductive technologies. Williams (1986) notes that while these technologies are completely female centered they are almost entirely male controlled. "It is amazing and frightening to contemplate the fact that most of the scientists who deal with women's reproduction belong to that half of the human race that does not menstruate, experience pregnancy, give birth or go through menopause" (p. 5).

3. The rise of medical authority and its power in defining a "normal" woman, largely based on patriarchal assumptions about women. Corea (1985) points out that medicine is a powerful means of social control particularly in terms of women. She points to abortion laws, contraception laws, cases of court ordered obstetrical intervention, prosecution of women for "fetal abuse," as well as the experiences of women in Romania as attempts to control women and their behavior. Koch and Morgall (1988) state, "as no technology is 'neutral' but basically a means of control of processes, and in this case human biological processes, control of technology gives control over lives—biopower, as Michel Foucault (1978) calls it" (p. 186).

4. The experimentation on women's bodies without full knowledge of the effects. Medicine has a very poor track record when it comes to women's health. DES, Depo-Provera, and the Dalkon shield are potent reminders of medicine's attempts to assist in controlling reproductive processes. Klein and Rowland (1989) identify major health concerns with the fertility drugs given to women involved

in IVF programs. Warren (1988) identifies this concern as the primary issue in terms of reproductive technologies. She questions "whether IVF is sufficiently beneficial to IVF patients to justify the commercial marketing of these procedures or even continued research and development" (p. 38). Success rates are low and are not depicted honestly. There is little discussion of the dangers from the drugs, superovulation, infection, and personal and psychological effects, including the disruption of work and relationships and the feelings of loss and failure.

With any discussion of experimental procedures the question of informed consent is raised. An even more fundamental question is related to why women participate in these procedures. A number of feminist researchers argue that women's reproductive choices are conditioned by the society in which they live and that "patriarchal society with its pronatalist ideology makes it difficult for women to make free choices" (Warren, 1988, p. 40).

5. Reproductive technologies reduce women to sources of eggs, embryos, and wombs and obliterate the value of women as autonomous beings (Hynes, as cited in Koch & Morgall, 1987, p. 182). Embryos become the focus. The associated developments of prenatal diagnoses and therapy serve to reinforce the separation of the woman and fetus. "The 'fetus-as-patient' mentality which often accompanies the new reproductive technologies endangers women's rights" (CRIAW, 1990, p. 5).

6. These technologies perpetuate the myth of fulfillment through motherhood. Hanmer (1987) and Rothman (1989), for example, argue that while some women's options may be increased with these technologies, they actually decrease options for many others by suggesting that women's lives are unfulfilled if they do not bear children and especially a child that is genetically linked to the parents.

Why do women want children so badly that they are willing to undergo the immense emotional, physical, and often financial costs of using one of these technologies? As Williams (1986) suggests:

The rush by doctors and scientists to provide expensive, invasive and traumatic "fix-it" technologies to help women bear children usually at great trauma and expense to themselves and often to society definitely serves to support the idea that childbearing is so important that it justifies the enormous degree of intervention and the huge cost associated with reproductive technologies. (p. 9)

7. The cost of the procedure skews health care resources and causes other areas, particularly research into the causes of and treatments for infertility, to receive much less attention. The World Health Organization estimates that for the cost of one live IVF baby, 100 women could be prevented from becoming infertile (CRIAW, 1990).
8. Concerns regarding the process of policy making in relation to reproductive technologies and who has access.

From this brief review of mainstream and feminist literature, important differences in the approach taken and the subsequent concerns identified appear. Similar, however, in both approaches is the lack of attention given to the role of the nurse in the processes involved in reproductive technologies.

The Role of the Nurse

As noted in the introduction, the nursing literature has generally approached reproductive technologies from a mainstream perspective that examines technological developments, ethical issues focusing on fetal versus maternal rights, or the ways nurses help couples cope with the processes involved in reproductive technologies. The lack of a specifically feminist voice here is clearly evident. A review of nursing journal articles published and listed in the CINAHL indexes since 1985 indicates that there are three general approaches extant. Articles were categorized into those dealing with ethical issues (Francis & Nosek, 1988; Mander & Whyte, 1985; Marmaduke & Bell, 1989; Poteet & Lamar, 1986; Shannon, 1990; White, 1988; Wright, 1989); with the technical aspects (Battle-Mutter, 1988; Creighton, 1985; Fincham, 1987; McLaughlin, 1989; Rabar, Falksohn, & Morton, 1988; Pace-Owens, 1985, 1989); and those articles dealing with the role of the nurse in helping couples cope with the IVF process (Frank, 1990; Frey, Stenchever, & Warren, 1989; Gaze, 1990; Kuczynski, 1989; Lovell, 1988 a, b; Milne, 1987; Olshanky, 1988). There are very few authors who take a more critical perspective (Sandelowski, 1988; Spallone, 1990); and one author examines the impact of IVF on women in particular (Stewart & Glaser, 1986).

Marmaduke and Bell (1989), for example, discuss the dilemmas surrounding IVF and embryo transfer. They raise questions related to the moral consideration of the embryo and to the selection of IVF candidates. Unfortunately, while they ponder the future role of nurses in relation to these technologies, they note, "We must be prepared to meet these challenges as we move into the future" (p. 28). This last comment suggests a willingness to participate in the ongoing development and implementation of reproductive technologies notwithstanding the general absence of considerations of such implications for women. In this regard, while Poteet and Lamar (1986) examine the issues surrounding artificial insemination, they also take a mainstream position by identifying as important such issues as donor selection and screening, record keeping, and the impact on the children conceived by artificial insemination. Particular concerns for women, such as health risks, commodification of women's bodies, and medical control of access and procedures, are not addressed.

Another interesting phenomenon in the nursing literature is the use of the "couple" as the research subject. Frank (1990), Pace-Owens (1989), and Milne (1987), in addressing the concerns of the "couple" as the primary issue, see the nurse's role as that of counselor. Pace-Owens notes "a sympathetic nurse coordinator will want couples to look back after a treatment cycle and say they were glad they tried the treatment" (p. 96). In addition, all three researchers viewed reproductive technologies as helpful. "In vitro fertilization offers increasing numbers of infertile couples the chance to achieve a pregnancy" (Milne, p. 351).

There are the small number of researchers, however, who have addressed reproductive technologies from a more critical and woman-centered perspective. Sandelowski (1988), in identifying the problem of reproductive technologies for nursing, notes that "reproductive technology, embodying a conceptual system that emphasises fragmentation and separation, is antithetical to the philosophical foundation of nursing practice which aspires to holism and connection" (p. 36).

In conclusion, there are significant issues that nurses have yet to fully examine in relation to reproductive technologies. Because we have been slow to develop a critical woman-centered perspective, nurses have remained generally outside the important discussions taking place in society about reproductive technologies. When examined in this light, it becomes clear that nurses need to understand these developments and to make their voices heard on these issues.·

COURT ORDERED OBSTETRICAL INTERVENTIONS

On May 20, 1987, at 2118 hours a representative of the British Columbia department of Family and Child services arrived at the Grace Maternity Hospital in Vancouver, British Columbia, Canada. He was accompanied by three police officers, two social workers, and a number of doctors from the hospital. Their task was to enforce an apprehension order for the purposes of emergency medical treatment. What is unusual in this case was that the subject of the apprehension order was a fetus and the emergency medical treatment was a caesarean section to which the fetus's mother, Rose, had not consented. Although Rose did eventually consent, verbally, to the surgery, apparently almost at the door of the operating room, the child was still taken into custody after the delivery. Rose later appealed the apprehension of her child. A provincial court judge refused Rose's appeal. The basis for his judgement is unclear. Counsel for the Superintendent of Family and Social Services may have persuaded the judge that Rose's past conduct and difficulties as a parent indicated that the child required ongoing protection. However, the provincial Supreme Court set aside that decision and granted custody to the biological mother. The Supreme Court judge found that the definition of "child" under the Family Service Act did not include the unborn fetus, and therefore the apprehension order had no basis in law. He noted that "Should it be lawful in this case to apprehend an unborn child hours before birth, then it would logically follow that an apprehension could take place a month or more before term. Such powers to interfere with the rights of women, if granted and if lawful, must be done by specific legislation and anything less will not do." (Re "Baby R," 1988, p. 248).

The presence of the police and social workers certainly emphasizes the objective of controlling Rose. As frightening as this scenario sounds, it is important to realize that it was not unique. A number of such apprehensions and other interventions have occurred in Canada and the United States. Kolder, Gallagher, and Parsons (1987), who have provided the most concise compilation of information regarding court ordered obstetrical interventions, discovered that interventions included cesarean sections, hospital detentions, and intrauterine transfusions. According to their research, 15 court orders for cesarean sections were sought in 11 states and were obtained in all except Maine. Three court orders were sought for hospital detention and two were obtained; three orders were requested for intrauterine transfusions, of which two were obtained. Their data indicate that in these cases 81 percent of the women were nonwhite, 44 percent were unmarried, and none were private patients. In addition to compiling this data, the investigators also investigated attitudes of physicians involved in maternal-fetal medicine toward court ordered obstetrical interventions.

Further information collected by Kolder, Gallagher, and Parsons (1987) is extremely revealing. Forty-seven percent of the physicians questioned thought that "mothers who refused medical advice and thereby endangered the life of the fetus should be detained in hospitals or other facilities so that compliance can be assured" (p. 1193). A large percentage of physicians (47%)

thought that appropriate reasons for obstetrical intervention should be expanded to include such things as not following a proper diet. Finally, 26 percent of physician respondents thought that state surveillance of women who did not seek medical care in the third trimester was acceptable, indeed, "advocated" (p. 1193).

As a result of these cases, an increasing amount of research and discussion is taking place, in a variety of disciplines, related to court ordered obstetrical interventions: in medicine (Field et al., 1988; Jessup, 1990); in law (Locke, 1987; Rhoden, 1986); in philosophy (Annas, 1988); and in social work (Holbrook, 1990; Maier, 1988). The mainstream literature addresses this issue in a very similar manner to the perspective taken with reproductive technologies. In other words, there is an attempt to balance the rights of the woman with the rights of the fetus. Feminist writers, however, have also turned their attention to this issue (Kolder, Gallagher, & Parsons, 1987; Field, 1989), and their approach differs because of its woman-centered focus.

Martha Field (1989) has examined the situation of court ordered obstetrical interventions and the development of fetal abuse legislation. She notes that while access to birth control and abortion have become legally recognized, that there is a movement that attempts to control women in other ways: as potential or actual child bearers. These attempts are exemplified in such measures as detention, surveillance, medical interventions, threat of criminal charges, and the threat of the apprehension of the woman's child at birth. Field (1989) states that "controlling women to protect their fetuses is using pregnancy to deprive women of the most basic rights" (p. 116), and that such a use of pregnancy to the detriment of women goes against the recent recognition of women, pregnant or not, as competent persons with the ability to make decisions. Advocates of these types of control view the fetus as having rights and as separate from the woman who bears it. While this scenario may seem far fetched, the work of Kolder, Gallagher, and Parsons (1987) and the increasing number of prosecutions under fetal abuse laws indicate that it is time to examine and discuss these developments.

Field (1989) suggests that such moves to control women during pregnancy, as noted above, may be a backlash against the rights won by women in relation to control of reproduction. When one examines in more detail the implications of these measures, it becomes clear that they are not so much designed to improve fetal outcomes (i.e., healthier babies), as they are designed to control women. "If the real goal is not control of women but protection of the child-to-be and creation of as healthy a newborn population as possible, then appropriate means are education and persuasion, free prenatal care and good substance abuse and rehabilitation programs available free of charge to pregnant women" (p. 125).

Again, as with reproductive technologies, neither the feminist or mainstream literature acknowledges the important role nurses play in enforcing such interventions. When reading the court documents related to the "Baby R" case, one would never know that there were nurses involved in the case. It was, however, nurses who were preparing Rose for the operating room. What did they think? How did they feel wheeling Rose toward the operating room knowing she was being forced to undergo a cesarean section? No mention of nurses is made; again, nurses are invisible. Again, the lack of a critical woman-centered perspective in nursing encourages nurses to remain silent and ignored.

In this context, nursing research literature presents only a dearth of information regarding the issues of concern here. Bushy, Randell, and Matt (1989), Kroll (1987), Rhodes (1990), Sise (1988), and Twomey (1989) are researchers in nursing who have addressed court ordered obstetrical interventions, however.

Sandelowski (1983) notes the disturbing tendency of nurses involved in reproductive care to distinguish between the pregnant woman and her fetus and of the nursing literature to "view pregnant women as vehicles to be acted upon by the nurse in the interests of the fetus" (p. 321). The literature review conducted for this paper reveals little progress since that time. Twomey (1989) is the only other author who presents a critical woman-centered perspective. The other researchers focus on the more mainstream ethical issues, and the discussion is based on fetal versus maternal rights. Given the enormous questions raised in terms of these measures, one wonders why there has been virtually no attempt to examine these issues, particularly from a feminist perspective within nursing. One possible explanation for this lack of discussion is the lack of an analysis that helps nurses understand the implications, for themselves and for their patients, of both reproductive technologies and court ordered obstetrical interventions.

A CRITICAL WOMAN-CENTERED ANALYSIS
FOR NURSING

Despite the fact that nurses play "essential and sometimes powerful roles" in the implementation of reproductive technologies (Williams, 1989, p. 80) and in implementing court ordered obstetrical interventions, nurses remain invisible in the mainstream and feminist discussions. Watson (1990), who recognizes this invisibility in nursing, notes, "Yet, for some unintelligible reason, the vast cadre of female health and human caring professionals (nurses) continue to be invisible" (p. 63) in relation to decision making in the health care system. From the literature review presented here it seems that part of our invisibility is related to our willingness to accept the developments in reproductive technology and the use of court ordered obstetrical interventions (at least in some circumstances). The problem of nurses' participation in medicine's enterprise has been documented by Ashley (1980), who states, "In maintaining a close and longstanding relationship to medicine, psychiatry, gynecology, psychology and many other male dominated groups in the health field which are based on the non-capacity to care for women, nursing has done great damage to itself. . . . Women in nursing have not begun to examine the destructive nature of these relationships" (p. 16).

As developments in reproductive health care continue, it is more and more important for nurses to voice, clearly and loudly, their concerns about reproductive technologies and court ordered obstetrical interventions. To do so, nurses need to develop a critical, woman-centered analysis of these developments. Fundamantal to such an analysis is an analysis of reproduction. Perhaps the most cogent analysis here is offered by O'Brien (1981). Herself a midwife, O'Brien, using a historical materialist approach, explains reproduction in terms of male and female reproductive consciousness. Male reproductive consciousness is one of alienation; men are alienated from their seed (never completely assured of their paternity), indeed alienated from history. It is a consciousness that lacks connection to the past and to the future. Female reproductive consciousness does not experience alienation. It is founded on being connected. A woman experiences her connection to the child, through the labor of birth she knows the child is hers. Through the process of birth she is connected to the past, her own birth, and those before and to the future through the life of her child.

Men, in an attempt to mediate their alienation, create institutions that seek to appropriate or control children and procreativity. The historical focus on the "superior procreative potential for a sanctified sperm" (O'Brien, 1981, p. 48), for example, is continued today in reproductive technologies where women's bodies become containers for the all-important male seed. Burfoot (1989), Hanmer (1987), and Brodribb (1986) have used O'Brien's ideas and applied them to an analysis of reproductive technologies. Hanmer warns that reproductive technologies cause women to experience the same "discontinuous experience men now have" (1983, p. 188). Brodribb sees the threat that reproductive technologies represent to women's reproductive consciousness and states, "an integrative understanding of birth does not see parturition as a technological event, children as commodities or women as suitcases" (1989, p. 410). Burfoot concludes that "science and medicine enable a new mysticism based on an ancient male reproductive consciousness still active in its attempts to appropriate female procreativity and to ensure male continuity" (1989, p. 60).

In conclusion, O'Brien offers a woman-centered analysis of reproduction that can help nurses analyze reproductive technologies and the associated developments of court ordered obstetrical interventions. It becomes clear that in many ways these developments are not new at all; rather, they are recent developments in a long history of attempts to control women's reproduction as an attempt to control women. As nurses, it is critical to understand the importance of questioning our role in this oppression. It is time to speak out loudly in support of women. As Sandelowski (1988) notes, "Reproductive technology is changing not only the experience of maternity but also the long standing bond between nurses and childbearing women" (p. 43).

As an alternative to nurses' participation in reproductive technologies and court ordered obstetrical interventions, nurses need to stand with women as much to reconstruct a joyful sense of childbearing and maternity as to point out the hypocrisy of government policy and fetal rights groups. If society wants healthy babies, it must be willing to support women's health and women's decisions in reproduction.

CONCLUSION

In this paper I have briefly examined nursing's response to the developments in reproductive technologies and the use of court ordered obstetrical interventions. From a review of the nursing literature in the past five years, it appears that nursing researchers have generally been slow to address these issues and when they have it has been from a mainstream position which does not recognize the particular importance these developments have for women. The fact that nurses have, generally, not examined these issues, or when they have done so, it has not been from a woman-centered or feminist position, has caused nurses to be virtually absent from any non-nursing discussion. This despite the fact that nurses do play very important roles in the support of and implementation of both reproductive technologies and court ordered obstetrical interventions. As a result, nurses remain outside critical discussions related to women's health, reproductive care, and indeed about the future of society itself. Nurses need to construct a feminist analysis of these developments and nurses' roles in them. The work of Mary O'Brien (1981), for one, offers extremely useful insights that could be developed into a critical woman-centred nursing analysis of reproductive technologies.

Nurses must intervene in this discussion. If we do not, we will continue to remain invisible.

DISCUSSION QUESTIONS

1. This paper raises several questions about the absence of a critical or feminist voice in nursing literature on reproductive technology. What factors may explain the absence of a feminist perspective in nursing discussions regarding reproductive technology?

2. How do you think this absence/silence is viewed by society? What is at stake in the invitation to nurses to find a feminist voice regarding this issue? If a feminist voice did emerge in nursing literature, what kinds of responses might be expected from (a) society, (b) other providers, and (c) nurses themselves?

3. Hagell occupies or speaks from a feminist standpoint in this paper and invites nurses in maternal child health practice to locate themselves in this standpoint as well. As you compare this paper to those of Henderson, Allman, and Thompson, consider the dilemmas of proposing such a standpoint for nurses. Can nurses locate and occupy a single woman-centered standpoint from which they can apprehend, advocate for, and intervene in the reproductive concerns of women? Do class, race, and sexual orientation split this standpoint? If no common feminist standpoint exists, what political agenda can nursing develop with regard to reproductive technology?

REFERENCES

Annas, G. (1988). She's going to die: The case of Angela C. *Hastings Center Report, 18*(1), 23–25.

Ashley, J. (1980). Misogyny in nursing: Implications for the politics for care. *Advances in Nursing Science, 2*(3), 3–22.

Battle-Mutter, P. (1988). Making babies through in vitro fertilization. *RN, 51*(11), 34–36.

Brahams, D. (1988). A baby's life or a mother's liberty: A United States case. *Lancet, 1*(8592), 1006.

Brodribb, S. (1986). Off the block and onto the pedestal? Motherhood, reproductive technologies and the Canadian state. *Canadian Journal of Women and the Law, 1*(2), 407–423.

Burfoot, A. (1989). The tenacity of the alchemic imagination. *Resources for Feminist Research, 18*(3), 57–61.

Bushy, A., Randell, P., & Matt, B. (1989). Ethical principles: Applications to an obstetric case. *Journal of Obstetrical, Gynecological, Neonatal Nursing, 18*(3), 207–212.

Canadian Research Institute for the Advancement of Women. (1989). *Reproductive technologies and women: A research tool.* Ottawa: Author.

Canadian Research Institute for the Advancement of Women. (1990). *Submission to the Royal Commission on New Reproductive Technologies.* Ottawa: Author.

Corea, G. (1985). *The mother machine: Reproductive technologies from artificial insemination to artificial wombs.* Toronto: Fitzhenry & Whiteside.

Corea, G. (1987). The reproductive brothel. In G. Corea (Ed.), *Man made women* (pp. 38–51). Bloomington: Indiana University.

Creighton, H. (1985). In vitro fertilization. *Nursing Management, 16*(4), 12, 14.

Ehrenreich, B., & English, D. (1979). *For her own good.* New York: Anchor.

Field, D., Gates, E., Creasy, R., Jonsen, A., & Laros, R. (1988). Maternal brain death during pregnancy: Medical and ethical issues. *Journal of the American Medical Association, 260*(6), 816–822.

Field, M. (1989). Controlling the woman to protect the fetus. *Law, Medicine and Health Care, 17*(2), 114–129.

Fincham, E. (1987). The gift of life . . . gamete intrafallopian transfer (GIFT). *Nursing Times, 83*(48), 51–53.

Firestone, S. (1979). *The dialectic of sex.* London: Women's Press.

Francis, G. R., & Nosek, J. A. (1988). Ethical considerations in contemporary reproductive technologies. *Journal of Perinatal and Neonatal Nursing, 1*(3), 37–48.

Frank, D. (1990). Factors related to decisions about fertility treatment. *Journal of Obstetrical, Gynecological, Neonatal Nursing, 19*(20), 162.

Frey, K. A., Stenchever, M. A., & Warren, M. P. (1989). Helping the infertile couple. Infertility workup. *Patient Care, 23*(10), 29–30.

Gaze, H. (1990). Infertility: The waiting game. *Nursing Times, 86*(18), 31–33.

Hanmer, J. (1987). Transforming consciousness: Women and the new reproductive technologies. In G. Corea (Ed.), *Man made women* (pp. 88–109). Bloomington: Indiana University.

Holbrook, S. M. (1990). Adoption, infertility and the new reproductive technologies: Problems and prospects for social work and welfare policy. *Social Work, 35*(4), 333–337.

Hubbard, R. (1987). Eugenics: New tools, old ideas. *Women & Health*, *13*(1/2), 225–235.

Indenrigsministeriet. (1984). *Fremskridets Pris*. Kobenhaven.

Jessup, M. (1990). The treatment of perinatal addiction. *Western Journal of Medicine*, *152*(5), 553–558.

Klein, R., & Rowland, R. (1989). Hormonal cocktails: Women as test sites for fertility drugs. *Women's Studies International Forum*, *12*(3), 333–348.

Koch, L., & Morgall, J. (1987). Towards a feminist analysis of reproductive technology. *Acta Sociologica*, *30*(2), 173–191.

Kolder, V., Gallagher, J., & Parsons, M. (1987). Court ordered obstetrical interventions. *The New England Journal of Medicine*, *316*(19), 1192–1196.

Kroll, D. (1987). The consequences of fetal rights. *Midwives' Journal*, *83*(7), 59–60.

Kuczynski, H. J. (1989). The holistic health care of couples undergoing IVF/ET. *Midwives Chronicle*, *102*(1212), 9–11.

Locke, N. (1987). Mother v. her unborn child: Where should Texas draw the line? *Houston Law Review*, *24*(3), 549–576.

Lovell, B. (1988a). In Vitro fertilization: The birth of Michael. *Nursing Times*, *82*(44), 29–30.

Lovell, B. (1988b). In Vitro fertilization: A way of hope. *Nursing Times*, *82*(44), 26–29.

Maier, K. (1988). Fetal rights vs. women's rights: A feminist social work perspective on the "Baby R" case. *Resources for Feminist Research*, *17*(3), 119–123.

Mander, R., & Whyte, D. (1985). Assisted reproduction: Setting the limits. *Midwifery*, *1*(4), 232–239.

Marmaduke, A., & Bell, S. (1989). In Vitro fertilization and embryo transfer dilemmas. *Nursing Forum*, *24*(3, 4), 24–28.

McLaughlin, M. (1989). Gamete intrafallopian transfer (GIFT): A treatment for infertility. *Midwives Chronicle*, *102*(1212), 23.

Milne, B. (1987). Couples experience with in vitro fertilization. *Journal of Obstetrical, Gynecological, Neonatal Nursing*, September/October, 347–352.

Moss, K. (1988). New reproductive technologies: Concerns of feminists and researchers. *Affilia*, *3*(4), 38–50.

Oakley, A. (1986). *The captured womb*. Oxford: Blackwell.

O'Brien, M. (1981). *The politics of reproduction*. Boston: Routledge & Kegan Paul.

Olshansky, E. F. (1988). Responses to high technology infertility treatment. *Image*, *20*(3), 128–131.

Ontario Law Reform Commission. (1985). *Report on human artificial reproduction and related issues* (vols. 1–2). Toronto: Ministry of the Attorney General.

Pace-Owens, S. (1985). In Vitro fertilization and embryo transfer. *Journal of Obstetrical, Gynecological, Neonatal Nursing,* (Supplement) November/December, 44s–48s.

Pace-Owens, S. (1989). Gamete intrafallopian transfer (GIFT). *Journal of Obstetrical, Gynecological, Neonatal Nursing,* 18(2), 93–97.

Pappert, A. (1988 February 6). In Vitro in trouble. *The Globe and Mail,* pp. A1–2.

Poteet, G., & Lamar, E. (1986). Artificial insemination by donor: Problems and issues. *Health Care for Women International,* 7, 391–399.

Queensland. (1984). *Report of the special committee appointed by the Queensland Government to enquire into the laws relating to artificial insemination, in vitro fertilization, and other related matters.* Queensland, Australia: Author.

Rabar, F. G., Falksohn, C. O., & Morton, S. (1988). Ultrasonographic transvaginal ovum retrieval: A new approach to in vitro fertilization. *Journal of the Association of Operating Room Nurses,* 48(1), 42–43.

Re "Baby R." (1988). *British Columbia Law Reports,* 237–248.

Rich, A. (1986). *Of woman born.* New York: Norton.

Rhoden, N. (1986). The judge in the delivery room: The emergence of court ordered cesareans. *California Law Review,* 74(6), 1951–2030.

Rhodes, A. M. (1990). Maternal liability for fetal injury? *Maternal-Child Nursing,* 15(1), 41.

Rothman, B. (1989). *Recreating motherhood.* New York: Norton.

Sandelowski, M. (1983). Perinatal nursing: Whose speciality is it anyway? *Maternal Child Nursing,* 8, September/October, 317–322.

Sandelowski, M. (1988). A case of conflicting paradigms: Nursing and reproductive technology. *Advances in Nursing Science,* 10(3), 35–45.

Shannon, T. (1990). Ethical issues involved in in vitro fertilization. *Journal of the Association of Operating Room Nurses,* 52(3), 627–628.

Singer, P., & Wells, D. (1984). *The reproduction revolution.* New York: Oxford.

Sise, C. B. (1988). Maternal rights versus fetal interests: An ethical issue with nursing implications. *Journal of Professional Nursing,* 4(4), 262–267.

Spallone, P. (1986). The Warnock Report: The politics of reproductive technology. *Women's Studies International Forum,* 9(5), 543–550.

Spallone, P. (1987). Reproductive technologies and the state: The Warnock Report and its clones. In P. Spallone & D. Seinberg (Eds.), *Made to order: The myth of reproductive and genetic progress.* London: Pergamon.

Spallone, P. (1990). Infertility: The cost of conception. *Nursing Times,* 86(18), 28–31.

Stewart, S., & Glaser, G. (1986). Expectations and coping of women undergoing in vitro fertilization. *Maternal Child Nursing Journal,* 83(48), 103–113.

Twomey, J. G. (1989). The ethics of in utero fetal surgery. *Nursing Clinics of North America, 24*(2), 1025–1032.

Warren, M. A. (1988). IVF and women's interests: An analysis of feminist concerns. *Bioethics, 2*(1), 37–57.

Watson, J. (1990). The moral failure of the patriarchy. *Nursing Outlook, 38*(2), 62–66.

White, G. B. (1988). Infertility and ethical policy. *Nursing Connections, 1*(3), 16–22.

Williams, L. (1986). *But what will they mean for women? Feminist concerns about the new reproductive technologies.* Ottawa: CRIAW.

Williams, L. (1989). The overlooked role of women professions in the provision of in vitro fertilization. *Resources for Feminist Research, 18*(3), 80–82.

Wright, J. E. (1989). Redefining familial reproduction in the 1980's. *Clinical Nurse Specialist, 3*(3), 154–155.

8

Is Woman Born or Made?
Female Gender Identity
and Women's Health

Dorothy J. Henderson

*I*s a woman born or made? Does female gender identity arise out of an innate awareness of biological femaleness or does it develop in response to social learning and cultural conditioning over the years of childhood? How individuals become aware of their gender and how that awareness influences their personality development, attitudes, and behavior has been a major focus of psychoanalytic theory. In addition, the concept of gender identity has been influential in defining what constituted psychological health in males and females. Psychological tests, for example, were designed to determine "healthy" adjustment of males and females to their "inherent" masculinity or femininity. Chesler (1972), Lundy (1987), and Paige (1973) have all pointed out that women's gender identity conflict is a basis for a number of women's health problems.

Several developments in psychological, psychoanalytic, and feminist theory have challenged the early concepts of gender identity. Specifically, efforts have been made to differentiate the internal response to anatomy from the external response to societal expectations in the environment. These distinctions have been useful in highlighting the many components of gender identity. Unfortunately, they have also created an artificial separation between the anatomical and sociocultural influences on the development of gender identity. In addition, these distinctions have led to the creation of a variety of terms such as *sexual identity, sex role identity, gender identity, core gender identity,* and *gender role identity.* These terms have been used inconsistently in addressing health issues since their development.

Nursing scholars and researchers have increasingly recognized the salience of gender identity in women's health. Yet conceptualizations in the nursing literature reflect the ambiguity of the terms elsewhere. In a study designed to measure gender role identity and self-concept in pregnant women, for example, Brouse (1985) used the sex role inventory to assess gender role identity. Brown and Woods (1984) used the same instrument to measure "traditionally described masculine and feminine characteristics."

For nursing, the question of female gender identity arises out of an attempt to understand how women's health behaviors and problems are related to being female—anatomically, psychologically, and sociopolitically. It also arises out of a lack of clarity concerning the concept of gender identity and its relationship to self-identity.

In this paper, I will address the question of gender identity in women. I will begin by tracing the historical development of the concept of gender identity (and related terms) since the time of Freud, looking specifically at the "born" versus "made" distinction. I will then compare the works of Chodorow, Flax, and MacKinnon in terms of their views of the development of female gender identity and its relationship to women's self-identity. Finally, I will suggest a new understanding of the concept of female gender identity that is drawn from feminist nursing perspective.

GENDER IDENTITY

Freud (1961/1925) was the first to attempt to explain the origins of gender identity (although Freud did not use those terms, but referred to sexuality instead). He believed that gender identity was a psychological response to the discovered anatomical differences between the sexes. He argued neither boys nor girls were aware of gender differentiation until around three or four years of age when both sexes discovered that boys had penises and girls did not. Until that time both males and females were primarily bisexual with a more masculine orientation.

It is interesting to note here that Freud, who has been criticized for believing that anatomy is destiny, actually pointed to an event that happened after birth—the awareness of the lack of a penis—as being responsible for the female's resulting psychology. Although at first this may seem a subtle distinction, it is critical to Freud's explanation of female psychology. According to Freud (1961/1936), the effect of penis envy contributes to women having greater amounts of passivity, narcissism, vanity, and shame than men. His explanation for these attributes is based on the female having to reconcile herself to not being what she had originally thought she was: a male. Freud acknowledges that it is difficult to distinguish the role that social learning plays in shaping the "psychical peculiarities of mature femininity." He states, however, that in the case of penis envy early infant development outweighs (and, in fact, sets the pattern for) the influence of later experience.

Freud, therefore, depicted masculinity as the more natural or primary state for both males and females before the age of three, and femininity as the developed state for females. Thus, Freud could be interpreted as believing that man is born while woman is made.

The first challenges to Freud's ideas about women came almost immediately from several of Freud's contemporaries (Adler, 1932; Horney, 1933; Jones, 1935; Thompson, 1964). Horney and Jones argued that masculinity is not the original state for females; rather, there is a primary femininity in females that is grounded in female biology and a vaginal awareness. Thus, female gender identity did not develop in the female out of the awareness of something lacking but out of an innate sense of something she had: a vagina.

Alternatively, two other contemporaries of Freud, Adler (1925) and Thompson (1964), argued that the sociopolitical environment of women's lives has a significant influence on the development of female gender identity. Adler points out that women's sense of inferiority results from the lack of power they are granted in a society dominated by males. Similarly, Thompson believes that prevailing cultural negativity toward women in general leads to a woman's lack of self-acceptance. She specifically points out the negative attitudes towards women's sexuality and body. These attitudes include a feeling that a woman's sexual life is not as important as a man's, a derogation of women's genitals, and an assumption that a woman's genitals are unclean because of the genital secretions of the female, including menstruation.

In these early opinions of Freud's contemporaries, we can find both sides of the woman born or made argument. Adler and Thompson can be seen as arguing for "woman made, not born"; on the other hand, Horney and Jones believe in women born, not made. Certainly in the case of Horney, such categorization is somewhat simplistic. In this context, Horney also argues strongly that penis envy in women exists but by way of their resentment of the power that males have in society and that the penis symbolizes.

In the mid-1960s, Horney and Jones's views were revived by Erikson (1964) and Kestenberg (1968), among others. Erikson supports the idea of "women born," asserting that the "ground-plan" of the bodily differences between males and females leads to innate psychological differences between the two sexes. Kestenberg expands on this view, arguing both males and females experience an innate inner-genital phase that is connected to the maternal.

At about the same time, a variation on the theme was introduced. Reversing Freud's assumption that masculinity is the natural state of both sexes, Stoller (1968) asserts that primary femininity is basic to both sexes and that it is males who need to become masculine through a process of dis-identification with their mothers.

Stoller (1985) developed his definitions of gender identity out of his clinical work as a psychiatrist, using analysis (in the psychoanalytic meaning of the term) to study the origins of gender behavior. More specifically, he developed his theories about normal gender identity in males and females by studying male transsexuals who sought him or other psychiatrists out for treatment. Stoller believes that these subjects demonstrate the "primary femininity" that is in all young boys but that is usually not evident in the normal developmental process. Thus, he generalized from his theories about abnormal male development to normal female development.

Stoller (1985) argues that gender identity is not based on any innate awareness of anatomy but rather on the child-rearing practices of the parents. These practices are gender specific, however, because they are based on the parents' perception of the child's anatomy and, therefore, gender. Thus, Stoller seemed to support the woman made, not born, perspective, except for the fact that he believed in primary femininity and might therefore be said to espouse the view that women are born and men are made.

As revisions were being made in the theories of gender identity, new terminology was being introduced in an attempt to differentiate the various dimensions of the phenomenon. Freud and his contemporaries discussed gender identity only in terms of sexuality, that is, femaleness or maleness, not femininity or masculinity; gender was not mentioned. Recognizing the importance of culturally prescribed behaviors and attitudes on the development of gender identity, Money, Hampson, and Hampson (1965) introduced the term *gender role*. Although Money intended the term to be inclusive of both sexual behaviors and sex role behaviors, a second term, *gender identity*, was soon being used to mean the internalized experience of being male or female. According to Person and Ovesey (1983), gender role came to mean the public expression of this experience.

A further specification was introduced by Stoller (1968) who originated the term *core gender identity*. He describes this as the "sense of one's sex . . . that is part of one's gender identity but not all of it" (Stoller, 1985, p. 11). Gender identity is seen by Stoller as encompassing a wider range of behaviors and as being influenced by object relations.

To further explain the relationship between core gender identity, gender identity, and gender role, Person and Ovesey (1983) suggest that the concept of gender identity is actually composed of two supporting concepts: core gender identity and gender role identity. They define core gender identity as Stoller does: "an individual's self-designation of biological femaleness or maleness" (p. 206). Gender role identity was defined as "an individual's self-evaluation of psychological femininity or masculinity" (p. 206).

Person and Ovesey (1983) also argue that Stoller's view of primary femininity in both males and females is as misguided as Freud's view of masculinity as primary. They suggest that there is no evidence that either masculinity or femininity is the primary state for both sexes and that normal core gender identity arises from sex of assignment (being labeled as male or female at birth) and child rearing. They assert that gender organizes sexuality and that there is no innate awareness of body involved in the development of core gender identity. Thus, falling in the social learning camp, they see woman made and man made.

With the introduction of the new concepts of gender role identity and core gender identity, Money, Hampson, and Hampson's original intent to recognize, but not separate, biology and psychology was sacrificed in an attempt for greater clarity. Such supposed clarity, however, has proved to be elusive. With greater theoretical "specificity" has come a reification of the split between the individual's psychological response to anatomy and an individual's psychological response to the meaning that society gives to gender.

The proliferation of terms does not stop with core gender identity and gender role identity, however. Other terms such as *sex role identity* and *sexual identity* can also be found. In addition, the meaning ascribed to any of the terms associated with gender identity is as dependent on the discipline and political opinions of the author as on the phenomenon being described.

Much of this effort at clarification has been an effort to maintain the distinction between that which is of the mind/culture and that which is of the body/nature. Thus, gender role identity and sex role identity refer to that which is culturally and psychologically shaped and known. Sexual identity and core gender identity refer to that which is given by nature and known, tacitly, in the body. And according to some theorists, such as Stoller, even core gender identity is known because it is taught, not because it is experienced bodily.

FEMINIST VIEWS ON GENDER IDENTITY

Psychoanalytic views on female gender identity have been a key focus of feminist critique since the beginning of the second wave of feminism in the early 1970s (Friedan, 1974; Millett, 1970; Hare-Mustin, 1983). At the same time, a psychoanalytic feminist theory has developed based primarily on the work of Chodorow (1978, 1989), with subsequent work by Miller (1986), Gilligan (1982), and Flax (1987, 1989). Although not a psychoanalyst, MacKinnon (1989) has also focused heavily on female sexuality and, indirectly, on female gender identity. How three of these theorists, Chodorow, Flax, and MacKinnon, address the concept of female gender identity will be compared in the next section.

According to feminist psychoanalytic theory, the development of the self cannot be separated from the development of a gender identity (Chodorow, 1989). In addition, the very concept of self in Western society cannot be separated from the issue of gender (Flax, 1990).

According to Chodorow's early work (1978), the very fact that women are the primary caretakers of both male and female children provides different developmental experiences for boys and girls. This results in men and women having different constructions of self and of their gender identity. A woman's early relationship with her mother allows her to develop a sense of self that is continuous and relational to others and to maintain flexible ego boundaries. In fact, Chodorow (1978) states that the "basic feminine self is connected to the world" (p. 169). She sees this as both a potential strength (enables intimacy) and a problem (threatens autonomy) for women's psychological development.

When compared with women, Chodorow (1978) continues, the psychological development of males primarily raised by women is quite different. Because men, at a young age, must definitively separate from their mothers in order to establish their masculine identity, they develop a sense of self that is separate and that is maintained by more rigid ego boundaries than that of women. Chodorow (1989) argues further that the asymmetry created when women are the primary parents leads to misogyny in both sexes; although more true in men, both males and females attempt to separate from the "powerful mother." For a boy this separation from the mother is accomplished by devaluing his mother and holding her and all things feminine (including his own femininity) in contempt. In contrast, a girl develops a hostility toward her mother that can lead to a sense of self-deprecation as she develops her own identity.

Chodorow's (1978) early work is clearly drawn from that of Stoller. Both describe the need for males to "dis-identify" from the mother, and both indicate, contrary to Freud's work, that it is the male that has the difficult gender (and self) identity development. Chodorow also seemed to support Stoller's view that gender identity and self-identity developed in response to parental attitudes and handling primarily. Unlike Stoller, however, Chodorow specifically pointed to gender asymmetry in parenting as being responsible for the differences in development between males and females. Thus, Chodorow's earlier work placed her in the social learning camp of woman and man made, with the female being somewhat closer to born than the male.

Originally focusing on the sociocultural influences on the development of gender and self-identity, Chodorow (1989) now suggests that feminist psychoanalytic theorists must revisit the views of those who believed in the innate awareness of female anatomy as contributing to gender identity. In terms of the relationship of core gender identity to gender role identity, Chodorow asks, "What is the extent to which female development is embedded in sexual difference and genital evaluation and experience: how does genital apprehension affect gender identity and sexuality?" (p. 193). In terms of the relation of gender identity and self-identity, Chodorow asks, "How important is gender identity, in the broadest sense, to women's sense of self? (p. 193). Although clearly not abandoning her sociological perspective, Chodorow seems to be acknowledging the need, as did Freud, to explore more thoroughly the meaning of the body to the mind.

From a different perspective and with a very different point of view, MacKinnon (1989) denies any links between the social meaning of being a woman and anatomical differences between the sexes. MacKinnon declares that gender socialization is the process of women coming to identify themselves as sexual beings that exist for men. She argues that in contemporary Western society male dominance defines female sexuality. She further argues that this sexuality dictates gender identity: males as dominant and females as submissive. Thus, according to MacKinnon, the female identifies her self as a submissive woman because of her unequal sexual relation to the male in a society where male dominance results in sexual and other violence toward women on a general scale. MacKinnon makes her position on the social construction of gender clear; she is in agreement with de Beauvoir, whom she quotes: "one is not born, one rather becomes a woman" (1989, p. 109).

MacKinnon's (1989) work is congruent with Chodorow's (1978) earlier work in that it views the female (as we can know her at this point) as made and not born. However, MacKinnon sees this creation of the female sense of self as originating in a culture that is completely male dominated. Chodorow focused more on the family and the female-as-mother as the root of female identity. Thus, while both Chodorow and MacKinnon offer sociological views of the development of female gender identity, MacKinnon's links to culture and society are more direct and explicit than Chodorow's.

In reading these two theorists, one develops a very different sense of what women and their reality is like. MacKinnon (1989) argues that any analysis of women's reality must recognize that it is male power that defines that reality. In this sense, it is not really possible now to know what being a woman would be like out from under male dominance. Being female is defined by oppression. Similarly, relatedness among women has nothing to do with having similar anatomies or with the shared experience of having been mothered by a female. According to MacKinnon, what women share is the experience of being treated like women: "Restrictions, conflicting demands, intolerable but necessarily tolerated work, the accumulation of constant small irritations and indignities of everyday existence . . ." (p. 85).

Chodorow (1978, 1989), on the other hand, sees a less bleak picture of female existence and identity in our society. She does offer a description of what women are like and suggests that identity development from her perspective has both positive and negative aspects for women. For example, she sees women as sharing more than a lived experience of oppression, proposing that they share a sense of relatedness to others. And in her more recent work, Chodorow (1989) seems to suggest that they may share a common meaning of being female anatomically as well.

A third voice in feminist theory, Flax (1987, 1989) seems to fall somewhere in between Chodorow and MacKinnon. In terms of self-identity and gender identity, Flax (1987) asserts that a woman's sense of gender and self are partially formed by her repression of her less socially acceptable selves, such as her sexual self and her autonomous self. She argues that in a male-dominated society the only self that is acceptable in women is the social self. She suggests further that the self develops out of one's gender identity rather than the reverse.

More recently, Flax (1989) asks similar questions to those of Chodorow (1989). Noting that the sex/gender dichotomy appears to stem from other "culture specific oppositions" like body/mind and nature/culture, Flax asks: "Does anatomy (body) have no relation to mind? What difference does it make in the constitution of my social experiences that I have a specifically female body?" (1990, pp. 147–148).

In summary, the analysis of MacKinnon as well as the questions of Flax and Chodorow must guide our future exploration of women and gender identity. We have needed the feminist critique of "anatomy is destiny," and we have benefited from understanding the social construction of gender. We have moved beyond the androcentric fallacy that woman is born. It is now time to move beyond the dualism implied in the belief that woman is made. This view denies the integration of the body/mind, implying that the body has no meaning beyond its immediate reality as a vehicle of existence. Surely the body informs the mind as the mind informs the body. What are the messages that are transmitted? What does it mean to a woman that she is in a female body and in an androcentric society?

This does not assume that the meaning of the body is independent of the socially constructed meaning of the body. But neither does it assume that there is no meaning to the body other than what has been socially constructed.

FEMALE GENDER IDENTITY FROM A FEMINIST NURSING PERSPECTIVE

The questions raised by feminist theorists are particularly relevant to the discipline of nursing. The integration of the body/mind and the interaction of the person and the environment are key concepts of many nursing theorists (Newman, 1986; Parse, 1981; Rogers, 1990). In addition, nursing's focus on the health of whole persons in their environment provides an appropriate framework for further exploration of the concept of gender identity. And nursing, unlike psychology, psychoanalysis, or even feminist scholarship, can be considered an "embodied" discipline. Nurses' experience and history of being physical caregivers makes them uniquely situated to contribute to this exploration.

A feminist nursing response to the question "Is woman born or made?" is to replace the "or" in that question with "and" and add "How" to the beginning. How is woman born and made? As nurses we need a new understanding of female gender identity that does not maintain the dichotomization of the body/mind and that acknowledges the relationship of gender identity and self-identity.

I suggest a new definition for female gender identity: "A tacit knowing and conscious awareness of self as woman through an integrated experience of one's anatomy, psyche, culture, and relatedness to other women." It is hoped that this definition can guide further inquiry into the question "How is woman born and made?" and can provide both greater depth and clarity to nursing research and practice in women's health.

DISCUSSION QUESTIONS

1. This paper problematizes the oppositions of mind/body and culture/nature, arguing that such dualistic thinking has made it difficult to sort out the meaning of gender identity. Why is it important for nurses to consider these questions?

2. In this paper, Henderson focuses on feminist revisions of object relations theory and presents these revisions as sociohistorical events that alter previous psychoanalytic work on gender identity. Although this paper does not include a review of Lacan's contributions to psychoanalytic theory, it does point in directions that are suggested by Lacan (see, for example, Tamsin, Lorraine, *Gender, identity and the production of meaning*, Westview, 1990). When Henderson asks the question "How is woman both born and made?" she is asking us to think about the production of meaning in culture as well as what role "tacit knowing in the body" plays in regard to gender and self-identity. How is gender identity "given" and "produced?" Why is it important for nurses to think about these questions?

3. Comparing this paper to those of Allman and Allen, think about the connections between the explanations or discourses that we use in nursing and the effect of these explanations or discourses on our practice. What sorts of explanations about gender will be adequate for nursing practice?

REFERENCES

Adler, A. (1932). *The practice and theory of individual psychology.* New York: Harcourt, Brace and Company.

Brouse, S. (1985). Effect of gender role identity on patterns of feminine and self-concept scores from late pregnancy to early postpartum. *Advances in Nursing Science, 7,* 32–47.

Brown, M., & Woods, N. (1984). Correlates of dysmenorrhea: A challenge to past stereotypes. *Journal of Gynecological Nursing, 259–266.*

Chesler, P. (1972). *Women and madness.* Garden City, NY: Doubleday.

Chodorow, N. (1978). *The reproduction of mothering: Psychoanalysis and the sociology of gender.* Los Angeles: The University of California Press.

Chodorow, N. (1989). *Feminism and psychoanalytic theory.* New Haven, CT: Yale University Press.

Erickson, E. (1964). The inner and the outer space: Reflections on womanhood. *Daedalus, 983, 582–606.*

Flax, J. (1989). *Thinking fragments: Psychoanalysis, feminism, and postmodernism in the contemporary west.* Berkeley: University of California Press.

Freud, S. (1961). Some psychical consequences of the anatomical distinction between the sexes. In J. Strachey (Ed. & Trans.), *The standard edition of the complete psychological works of Sigmund Freud* (Vol. 19, pp. 248–258). London: Hogarth Press. (Original work published 1925.)

Freud, S. (1961). Femininity. In J. Strachey (Ed. & Trans.), *The standard edition of the complete psychological works of Sigmund Freud* (Vol. 22, pp. 112–135). London: Hogarth Press. (Original work published 1936.)

Friedan, B. (1974). *The feminine mystique.* New York: Dell.

Gilligan, C. (1982). *In a different voice: Psychological theory and women's development.* Cambridge, MA: Harvard University Press.

Hare-Mustin, R. (1983, May). An appraisal of the relationship between women and psychotherapy: 80 years after the case of Dora. *American Psychologist, 593–601.*

Horney, K. (1933). The denial of the vagina, a contribution to the problem of genital anxieties specific to women. *International Journal of Psychoanalysis, 14, 57–70.*

Jones, E. (1935). *Early female sexuality. Papers on psychoanalysis.* Boston: Beacon Press.

Kestenberg, J. (1968). Outside and inside, male and female. *Journal of the American Psychoanalytic Association, 16, 457–520.*

Lundy, C. (1987). Sex-role conflict in female alcoholics: A critical review of the literature. *Alcoholism Treatment Quarterly, 4, 69–78.*

MacKinnon, C. (1989). *Toward a feminist theory of state.* Cambridge, MA: Harvard University Press.

Miller, J. B. (1986). *Toward a new psychology of women.* (2nd ed.). Boston: Beacon Press.

Millet, K. (1970). *Sexual politics.* Garden City, NY: Doubleday.

Money, J., Hampson, J. G., & Hampson, J. L. (1965). Sexual incongruities and psychopathology: The evidence of human hermaphroditism. *Bulletin of Johns Hopkins Hospital, 98, 43–57.*

Newman, M. (1986). *Health as expanding consciousness.* St. Louis: Mosby.

Paige, K. (1973, September). Women learn to sing the menstrual blues. *Psychology Today,* 41–46.

Parse, R. (1981). *Man-living-health: A theory for nursing.* New York: John Wiley.

Person, E., & Ovesey, L. (1983). Psychoanalytic theories of gender identity. *Journal of the American Academy of Psychoanalysis, 11,* 203–226.

Rogers, M. (1990). Nursing: Science of unitary irreducible human beings: Update 1990. In E. Barrett (Ed.), *Visions of Rogers' science-based nursing* (pp. 5–11). New York: National League for Nursing.

Stoller, R. (1968). *Sex and gender.* New York: Science House.

Stoller, R. (1985). *Presentations of gender.* New Haven, CT: Yale University Press.

Thompson, C. (1964). In M. Green (Ed.), *Interpersonal psychoanalysis: The selected papers of Clara M. Thompson.* New York: Basic Books.

9

Language and the Reification of Nursing Care

Akemi Hiraki

INTRODUCTION

In this paper, I will focus on the meaning of language and its centrality in the transformation of nursing practice. From a critical hermeneutics perspective, language is viewed as a medium in which human beings participate in their world. According to Ricoeur (1983), language as medium can disclose as well as conceal the meanings of human experience. I will argue that the language of nursing practice gives legitimacy to a technical rationality that creates conditions for the reification of the human experience of nursing care. My premise here is that the nursing process as a problem-solving method, when inappropriately applied, has the power to decontextualize the nurse-patient relationship, work as a tool of institutional control, and perpetuate a technocratic ideology that is patriarchal in nature.

Sections of this chapter are reprinted from *Advances in Nursing Science*, Vol. 14, No. 3, pp. 9–11, with permission of Aspen Publishers, Inc. © 1992.

As concept, nursing process derives from an analytical-empirical scientific tradition. In the past 25 years, nursing education has attempted to standardize the concept of nursing care in its curricula, hoping to secure nursing's professional integrity. This was done by defining the organization of nursing care as a scientific problem-solving approach called nursing process. Inherent in this approach is the notion of observable data and predictable outcomes. Nursing care is evaluated as effective when measurable, expected outcomes result from the planned action within the problem-solving methodology. Kobart and Folan (1990) state that this reductionistic rationality, common to medical science, is based on a male worldview of what knowledge is. The authors suggest that nursing's attempt to break from the paternalistic influence of medicine to become an autonomous profession has lead to defining "itself in medicine's own image" (p. 310). Such reductionistic rationality is particularly valued in nursing education because of its perceived scientific, value-free nature and is, therefore, used extensively throughout nursing curricula. Nursing process, as its exemplar, is used as an organizing structure in the belief that nursing process can mediate theory and practice.

In her argument against the idea of a value-free science, Botha (1989) describes a nursing paradigm as a group commitment to a framework of beliefs about the world. These paradigms are sanctioned commitments to interpreting data in a certain way based on the consents and convictions of a scientific nursing community. These paradigms act as models to explain reality but should not be interpreted as "the" reality. In her critique, Botha contends that a reductionist attitude prevails and is perpetuated through education to new generations of nurses "who are initiated in a relatively dogmatic way into a pre-established problem-solving tradition" (p. 50).

Let me clarify here that I do not advocate eliminating this method of problem solving within nursing practice. Certainly, there are areas of practice where this way of thinking is appropriate and needed. For example, in the technical skills of physical care of the patient, my argument centers on encouraging nurses to reconsider the power that language has on the everyday reality of their practice. When nursing process, as a method of problem solving, oversteps its boundaries and becomes a metaphor for nursing care, it redescribes the reality of the nurse-patient relationship in ways that we may not have intended.

Numerous discussions prevail in the nursing community about the core values guiding nursing practice, with language as a focus for analysis. From a hermeneutics stance, the act of speaking is a learning process that can effect or prohibit transformations in nursing practice. Since human experience is linguistically mediated and situated within a historical and social world, it follows that for nursing theory to be authentic, it must also be situated in the everyday life of the practicing nurse. When nursing theory and practice are dialectically involved, contraditions about theory or practice can be made problematic, and new meanings renegotiated.

Myra Levine (1989) contends that the ethics of practice are concealed or revealed in the language that describes nursing activity. She cautions against readily following fashions in language, which nurses have a tendency to do, without carefully reflecting on how language affects nursing's overall mission. Words taken from the marketplace, for example, to describe the recipient of nursing care as *consumer* or the modeling of clinical diagnostic language after medicine take unexpected turns. Though the intent of developing the nursing diagnosis was to provide a precise language for practice, Levine argues that the language of nursing diagnosis is a private language among nurses that gives no meaningful information to other health providers. On the other hand, medical diagnoses are useful information for nurses. Should not nursing diagnoses be useful information for physicians as well?

For Watson (1990), the development of nursing knowledge that encourages the view of humans and health caring processes as problems to diagnose gives power to these problems by according them law like status, separate from the experiences of human beings. From this perspective, nursing care results in technical and mechanical approaches. Watson describes knowledge that lacks self-reflection and critique as a "formula approach to people, objectifying, codifying, and reifying human experiences with 'official knowledge' that takes on a life of its own—a life that is separate, decontextualized, rather than connected" (p. 19).

Reification of nursing care refers to the ways that social institutions such as education, health care, and government have legitimized the objectification of nursing care. Reification is the transformation of social relations from relations between persons to relations between things. It is historically transient and characteristic of commodity production, especially of capitalist society. Accordingly, there is a depersonification of human beings and a personification of things. Human activity becomes a derivative of prevailing conditions and is reduced to noncreative functions. A person is no more than a performer of a ready-made role, a functional means of producing things. Reification is a socially necessary illusion—both accurately reflecting the reality of the capitalist exchange process and hindering its cognitive penetration (Heid, 1980).

LANGUAGE AND THE SOCIAL CONSTRUCTION OF NURSING PRACTICE

Ricoeur's interest lies in the inventiveness of language despite the objective limits and codes that govern it. He believes that despite technologic and political interests that obscure the diversity and potentiality of everyday language, it is possible to rejuvenate the metaphorial and narrative function of language for the benefit of all forms of language usage (1979). Although nurses are immersed in the technological language that prevails in health care institutions, there are spaces in their everyday conversations where possibilities arise to thematize the contradictions in language that arise in their practice. These events are possible because of the metaphorical characteristic of language.

The function of metaphor and its implication for interpretation is, for Ricoeur, a redescription of reality. Ricoeur (1979) believes that the power of metaphor lies in its referential function and its potential for creating new meanings within a specific context. Accordingly, possibilities of meanings are created when metaphors contradict or disrupt the literal use of words or phrases, thereby transforming the sense of the term and its referential meaning.

As a metaphor, the polysemous feature of "nursing process" presents a paradox in the sense that the "process" suggests an interactive mode of care. By definition, however, nursing process is a very specific problem-solving method informed by what Habermas (1976) would term a *technical interest*. Any possible interactive communication is by the nature of this rationality secondary to the "rules" of the method.

Swedish educators Lundh, Soder, and Waerness (1988), concerned that Swedish nursing education was uncritically adopting American nursing theories into their curriculum, critiqued nursing process. This critique from educators outside American culture is quite revealing. They found, for instance, that the nursing process model is similar to descriptions of various planning models and research processes, especially those for medical decision making. Unlike the other models, "nursing process" does not have specific technological or biological aspects within it; rather, it maintains focus on relationships with people. According to Habermas's cognitive interest theory, it is appropriate for instrumental rationality to inform technical actions that control our natural world. But when instrumental actions affect the social life of people, instrumental rationality exceeds its boundaries. For Habermas (1976), decisions about the practical life of individuals and society must be made discursively among the people affected, within a domination-free situation. If dialogue is not possible, then the authority of science is left unquestioned and sets up the possibility for an oppressive context.

A metaphor's power lies in its possibility of uncovering the contradictions that arise when one area of human cognitive interest extends into other areas of social life. Lundh, Soder, and Waerness (1988) found that nursing process in American nursing theories could be interpreted in two ways. First, nursing process is what actually happens when one provides nursing care. The authors contend that many nurses would disagree with this interpretation because nursing care is more than instrumental rationality and that "good nursing" can be based on premises other than those of calculative reasoning.

Second, nursing process is a normative model of what should be performed. From this viewpoint, nursing process may not be an accurate description of how nursing is actually performed, but it might be a useful description of what "ought" to be. The use of the nursing process model by nurse licensing bodies and professional accreditation organizations to set standards of practice attests to the normative application of this way of thinking. Lundh, Soder, and Waerness (1988) caution against the unconscious normative use of the nursing process model as a standard that contributes to the "scientification of nursing." They contend that this approach has the risk of distancing the nurse from the immediacy of the nurse-patient relationship by objectifying the patient's experiences.

Lundh, Soder, and Waerness (1988) argue that nursing theories, rather than reflecting what happens in practice, are often normative models of conduct; that is, they address how nursing should be practiced.

> In the Swedish debate it has become usual to argue that they are not really theories but models. That is, they specify certain rules for action that should be followed in nursing work. This modesty is, however, rarely shared by the American examples. These are held to be not only a normative ideal but also a description and explanation of what happens in nursing relationships (p. 38).

Lundh, Soder, and Waerness (1988) believe that the contradictions in the American nursing theories are not readily seen by most American nurses. They conclude their argument by emphasizing the possibility of patient domination if these theories are not questioned and reinterpreted. They believe that nurses have a moral responsibility to promote patient autonomy and self-understanding rather than participate in the oppressive relationships that could emerge if nursing theories are left unchallenged.

Nursing process, as instrumental action, follows a set methodology of assessment, diagnosis, planning, implementation, and evaluation based on measurable outcomes. The technical interest informing nursing process disallows the possibility of appropriately addressing the practical questions inherent in nursing care since the aim of this cognitive interest is control and predictability. When instrumental rationality is used to solve practical problems, power is manifested as domination and coercion. There is more to a nurse-client relationship than instrumental action.

Rew and Barrow (1987) conducted a study of intuition used in nursing practice. These investigators found that nurses relied on intuition as part of the decision-making process. Be that as it may, with the increasing legitimation of scientific thinking in nursing, there was a loss of credibility about the intuitive knowledge that was gained in the closeness of the nurse-patient relationship. The difficulty of articulating the intuitive experience is another contributing factor that has interferred with the development of intuitive knowledge.

Other authors, such as Chapman (1976) and Clark (1986), view nursing practice as essentially an interactive process between the nurse and patient within a social and cultural context. The complexity of the social reality is evidence for Clark to support multiple ways of viewing the world rather than the unitary view imposed by the empirical-analytic sciences. Clark argues for a reinterpretation of nursing actions with the view of human beings as self-determining and responsible for their own actions.

In his thesis on theory and practice in a highly advanced industrial society, Habermas (1973) states that science, technology, industry, and administration are intimately connected and that the laws of self-reproduction demand a continually escalating scale of technical control over nature and human organizations. In this situation, social institutions like our health care system, to maintain their self-reproductive capabilities, employ science for its powers of technical control.

Rather than viewing the everyday problems of practice and theory as issues for dialogue within the community of nurses, metaphors such as "system," "behavioral objectives," and "contralization" reify the social institutions of health care services and nursing education. Solutions to a "system" dysfunction or problem are characterized by the nurse or client "adapting" in such a way that the system regains its balance. Nursing process as a technical tool lends itself to technological solutions for problems such as fiscal management, the nursing shortage, or utilization of services. Nursing process also accommodates easily into the computerization of nursing care plans, checklist charting, and standardized or preprinted nursing care plans. This technocratic worldview, in which alternate solutions are rarely considered, is perpetuated by dominant relations continually reconstituting themselves by our everyday actions in our local areas of life. The political and economic pressures are not vague abstractions separate from us but are routinely reenacted in our social interactions. Nursing process, though a technical tool, is not neutral in its application.

CONCLUSION

The practical intent of critical hermeneutics is to overcome relations of domination and to realize that conditions of professional autonomy are informed by action-orienting self-understanding among nurses in a shared culture. We, in the nursing community, and from a critical stance, must participate in the social construction of our profession. Professional autonomy depends on nurses recovering the power to produce, distribute, and transform the meaning of nursing care.

DISCUSSION QUESTIONS

1. This paper raises questions about the function of language in nursing practice. For Hiraki, there is a place both for the problem-solving, instrumental aspects of nursing process and for the creative, metaphorical aspects of nursing process. What does she mean by instrumental action and technocratic interpretations of nursing process? What other (metaphorical) interpretations of nursing process does she invite us to consider?

2. What concerns do Swedish nurses have about nursing theory? Are these concerns shared by nurses in America?

3. In comparing this paper with those of Allen and Turkoski, we notice ways in which nursing discourse has reified the practice of nursing through its explanations, its theories, and its professional ideology. Can this be avoided? What other possible directions are suggested by these papers?

REFERENCES

Allen, D. (1985). Nursing research and social control: Alternative models of science that emphasize understanding and emancipation. *Image, 19*(2), 58–64.

Botha, M. E. (1989). Theory development in perspective: The role of conceptual framework and models in theory development. *Journal of Advanced Nursing, 13*, 49–55.

Chapman, C. M. (1976). The use of sociological theories and models in nursing. *Journal of Advanced Nursing, 1*, 111–127.

Clark, M. (1986). Action and reflection: Practice and theory in nursing. *Journal of Advanced Nursing, 11*, 3–11.

Habermas, J. (1973). *Theory and practice* (John Vertel, Trans.). Boston: Beacon Press.

Habermas, J. (1976). *Communication and the evolution of society* (T. McCarthy, Trans.). Boston: Beacon Press.

Held, D. (1980). *Introduction to critical theory.* Berkeley: University of California Press.

Kobart, L., & Folan, M. (1990). Coming of age in rethinking and the philosophies behind holism and nursing process. *Nursing & Health Care, 11*(6), 308–312.

Levine, M. E. (1989). The ethics of nursing rhetoric. *Image, 21*, 1, 4–6.

Lundh, U., Soder, M., & Waerness, K. (1988). Nursing theories: A critical view. *Image, 20*(1), 36–40.

Rew, L., & Barrow, E. (1987). Intuition: A neglected hallmark of nursing knowledge. *Advances in Nursing Science, 10*(1), 49–62.

Ricoeur, P. (1979). *The rule of metaphor.* Toronto: University of Toronto Press.

Ricoeur, P. (1983). *Hermeneutics and the human sciences* (J. Thompson, Trans.). London: Cambridge University Press.

Ricoeur, P. (1984). *Time and narrative* (K. McLaughlin & D. Pelleur, Trans.). Chicago: University of Chicago Press.

Thompson, J. B. (1981). *Critical hermeneutics: A study in the thought of Paul Ricouer and Jurgen Habermas.* Cambridge: Cambridge University Press.

Watson, J. (1990). Caring knowledge and informed moral passion. *Advances in Nursing Science, 13*(1), 15–24.

10

The Drive for Professionalism in Nursing: A Reflection of Classism and Racism

Sally O'Neill

In our society, women have lived and have been despised for living, the whole side of living that includes and takes responsibility for helplessness, weakness, and illness, for the irrational and the irreparable, for all that is obscure, passive, uncontrolled, animal, unclean—the valley of the shadow, the deep, the depths of life. All that the Warrior denies and refuses is left to us and the men who share it with us and therefore, like us, can't play doctor, only nurse, can't be warriors, only civilians, can't be chiefs, only Indians. Well, so that is our country. The night side of our country. If there is a day side to it, high sierras, prairies of bright grass, we only know pioneers' tales about it, we haven't got there yet. We're never going to get there imitating Macho-man. We are only going to get there by going our own way, by living there, by living through the night in our own country (Le Guin, 1989, pp. 116–117).

On the surface, the drive for professionalism by nursing has been fueled by the desire to increase nursing's standards of care and to obtain autonomy and respect from the public and other health care workers. Unfortunately, the model of professionalism nursing emulated was utilized by the dominant power in health care: medicine. This model, while ostensibly promoting quality control, worked to restrict entry to the medical "profession" to white, middle-class, and owning-class males (Ehrenreich, 1975). This restriction by class, race, and gender led to a profession that, with the enthusiastic support of hospital administrators and legislators, controlled and controls health care. Because of its success, the medical profession provided a model for other occupational groups, such as nursing.

The effect of following the medical model has led to the incorporation of aspects inherent to that model within nursing, namely, classism and racism. In order to analyze the connection between the drive for professionalism and classism and racism, I will contrast the characteristics of a profession with the process of professionalization as followed by medicine. I will then examine separately the effects on nursing of the classism and racism as embodied in the medical model. Classism and racism interlock and operate together in playing on nurses' fears of the stereotypes of becoming "powerless," unintelligent, or "lazy" as provided by the dominant culture of working-class women and women of color. Examining them separately will aid in this analysis. The effects of the mixed class makeup of nursing and subsequent conflicts caused by nursing's leaders owning-class (often called the upper class) and middle-class background will be discussed. Racism's effects will be described both in terms of the burdens caused to nurses of color and in terms of the loss to nursing of strategies used by African-American nurses to obtain goals. Finally, a conceptualization of nursing as a working-class profession is offered to resist the professional model provided by white, owning- and middle-class, male medicine.

The model for obtaining professional status for occupational groups came from medicine's movement toward professionalization throughout the late 1800s and early 1900s and culminating in the Flexner report of 1910. This report solidified medicine's public aims to upgrade itself from an unregulated craft to a regulated profession complete with standards of education and practice. Professional characteristics were championed so as to set standards of education, to control the scope of practice, and to regulate the quality of practitioners. In reality, however, the move to professionalization by male occupations in the late 1800s and early 1900s meant exclusionary regulations that increased their control over economics and maintained racial, gender, and class discrimination. After the Flexner report, medical schools restricted entry to white males from the owning and upper middle class. With the achievement of professional status, medicine consolidated its power over health care with its inherent sexism, racism, and classism.

With entry into medicine based on a four-year accredited medical school program and financial aid to enter medical school not available, working-class people were generally excluded from the profession. Since medical schools that educated women and people of color were not accredited and accredited schools did not admit women or people of color, the profession became white, male, owning and upper middle class (Ehrenreich & English, 1973; Ehrenreich, 1975, 1989; Woods, 1981; Reverby, 1987). This model, however, was a seductive one for nursing. It appeared to promise a pathway to achieving legitimacy, power, and autonomy.

During this same period (late 1800s to early 1900s), nursing leaders also attempted to standardize educational systems, to have state registration of nurses, and to define the scope of nursing practice. In 1920, the Goldmark report (in Reverby, 1987) on the state of nursing was published to provide a basis for nursing to achieve—through educational standards—what the Flexner report had achieved for medicine. However, the Goldmark report expressed an additional emancipatory aim: the separation of nursing schools from hospital control. In response to the report, medicine and hospital administrators indicated that although separation from hospitals and upgrading of facilities was good for medicine, it was not thought necessary for nursing. Lacking analyses based on class, race, and gender, but aware of the success achieved by medicine, nursing leaders continued to follow the medical model of professionalism.

It is important to remember here that while nursing ignored analyses based on feminism, class, and race, nursing also lacked political and economic power. Nursing leaders, unable to vote because of their gender and uninvolved themselves in the suffrage movement, expected male legislators to aid them in obtaining professional goals. Legislation that established registration of nurses, however, was not won easily. The New York state nursing registration experience is a pertinent example. Male legislators had to be persuaded to propose and support such a bill. Powerful opposition from medicine and hospital administrators appeared. What was deemed appropriate for male medicine was not seen as appropriate for female nursing (Tomes, 1983). At the time, nursing did not have access to financial resources of its own and often did not have access to foundations to the same extent that medicine did. The Flexner report, for example, was funded by the Carnegie Foundation. When the Carnegie Foundation was approached by nursing leadership to support the same kind of report, it turned them down. Although the Goldmark report was finally funded by the Rockefeller Foundation, its suggestions for implementation were not funded with the same largess as the Flexner report (Krampitz, 1987; Reverby, 1987).

CLASSISM AND NURSING

To understand what has happened to nursing pertaining to class issues, it is useful to view it in terms of classism operating within nursing. The term *classism* is defined here in a twofold manner: (1) as stereotyping on the basis of class with resulting discrimination and (2) as valuing class-based models, goals, and strategies from the dominant culture over those of groups peripheralized in the society. In the United States, the dominant cultural image has been of white owning- and middle-class males, while women, working-class people, and people of color have been disempowered and peripheralized (hooks, 1984). Hooks, in fact, critiques U.S feminism as being dominated by white middle-class women who look to the model of power provided by white middle-class males. This model, as prevalent as it is, continues to devalue the parenting and nurturing roles of women while valuing dominance over empowerment. In addition, it conveniently ignores the needs of the working class and the poor, such as earning a living wage in relation to the state of the economy as a whole, the necessity of public child care, and the necessity of provisions for adequate housing.

When viewed from a class analysis, nursing has also been stratified into leaders with owning- and middle-class goals and backgrounds and staff nurses who are further stratified into baccalaureate degree nurses, associate degree nurses, and diploma degree nurses (Woods, 1981). Such stratification can be partly explained as originating in the general exclusion of women from jobs other than nursing, teaching, secretarial work, or factory work. The resulting overcrowding of classes by women seeking professional status or the mixing of several classes as a result of overcrowding did not work to nursing's benefit. Without utilizing a class analysis that explained the mix of classes in nursing and the multiple needs of women in nursing, nursing leaders with few exceptions were prey to the seduction of the dominant model of power in society.

Beginning with Florence Nightingale's idea of "lady nurses" as superintendents and continuing in U.S. nursing with divisions between diploma, associate degree, and baccalaureate degree nurses, nursing has suffered from class divisions and their attending stereotypes. Although women entering nursing have been from all classes, values attributed to middle- and owning-class women were encouraged and required in all nurses. Deportment and "good character," for example, were not only indicative of femininity, but also of class. Women from working-class backgrounds provided qualities such as "hard working" and would become "good staff nurses," but only white, middle-class women, or women exemplifying that stereotype, would be appropriate for superintendents. In fact, until recently entry to and success in nursing schools has been limited both from economic inequities and class emphases such as character and deportment references (Muff, 1982; Reverby, 1987).

Although gains in independent status for nursing have been made through the move to separate schools of nursing from hospitals, avenues of entry into nursing have generally been closed off to women from working-class and economically deprived backgrounds. Educational programs that require four years of time as a student without financial and educational support create barriers for people from other than white middle-class and owning-class backgrounds.

Applying hooks's (1984) analysis to nursing, it is apparent that nursing also has been affected by classism. Strategic decisions made by nursing leaders who lacked an analysis based on class or on feminism meant that achieving professional status was seen as a more successful and more appropriate goal than that of agitating for better wages, better hours, and control over the allocation of nursing knowledge and skills. Goals common to all nurses have thus been separated into professional goals and working conditions. According to Allen (1987), the idea of being a professional has operated by appealing to the classism in nursing and by separating nurses from a possible source of strategizing and power. This separation has led to conflict between staff nurses, union nursing leaders, academic nursing leaders, and organizational leaders. As Baumgart (1983) and Gilchrist (1987) report, two Canadian nursing leaders, alliances between trade unions and professional organizations expand nursing's base of power. It is possible for both professional organizations and nursing unions to agitate for issues ranging from salaries to client-staff ratios.

RACISM AND NURSING

Black women in nursing have continually faced discrimination in terms of pay inequity, stereotypes, limited access to education, limited advancement, and restrictions in membership in nursing organizations. Professionalization in nursing did not mean increased opportunities for these nurses. The Goldmark report, however beneficial for nursing as an identifiable and unique profession, in recommending increased education for nurses, still meant increased burdens for black nursing. For example, in the South, it meant battling state registration laws that would not allow black nurses to be registered. Throughout the United States, standardization of educational requirements did not mean support to aid black nursing school facilities in meeting those requirements; it meant the closing of such nursing schools. It also did not mean reversing the very limited admission of blacks into better equipped and accredited white nursing schools (Harris, 1986/87; Hine, 1989). In this way, it replicated the effects of the Flexner report on the racial composition of medical schools.

PROGRESSIVE MODELS

In nursing, white racism and classism has resulted in the loss of emancipatory models of change provided by black nurses and working-class nurses of all colors. Black nurses and union nurses have acknowledged far more complexities and sites of coalition and resistance than are addressed by professionalizing strategies alone. In following the professional model of medicine with its unacknowledged racism and classism, nursing also perpetuated the racism and classism of the society around it and has been isolated from alliances that could provide models of strength.

Black nurses, however, in recognizing the racism of white nurses, have confronted it by organizing professional organizations specific to black nurses, by maintaining their alliances with black women's clubs, national black organizations, and black newspapers, and by fund raising from white philanthropic organizations. As evidenced by the written goals of the National Association of Colored Graduate Nurses (NACGN), the strategies of black nurses were both traditionally professional and designed to combat racism. The NACGN was established in 1908 with the goals of increasing educational standards and breaking down barriers for black nurses in education and on the job, as well as supporting black nursing leadership. In 1951, as black nursing leaders had achieved successes in ANA memberships and in increased admission of blacks to white nursing schools (Staupers, 1951), the NACGN was disbanded. In 1972, however, a group of black nurses led by Dr. Lauranne Sams organized the National Black Nurses Association (NBNA) to further combat racism. The NBNA was organized to support black nursing leadership and to address the health needs of the black community. By addressing the racism in both white nursing and in the society at large, the NBNA remains a model for nurses of assertive change.

Black nurses have not only relied on professional organizations for strength. Maintaining relationships with black women's social clubs supplied emotional, economic, and political support. Alliances between NACGN and black organizations, such as the NAACP and the Urban League, provided increased avenues for black nursing students to challenge discriminatory practices by white nursing schools. Finally, white philanthropic organizations became sources of needed funds for black nursing schools.

Models for progressive change have also been provided by collective nursing actions. For example, nurses in Denver, Colorado, brought the first comparable worth suit based on sex discrimination against the city of Denver. They contended that nurses, a primarily female occupation, were being paid less than city garbage collectors, a primarily male occupation.

Along with traditional labor concerns such as salaries and benefits, what could be considered as "professional" concerns have been achieved through bargaining. Beginning in 1986 and successfully ending in 1988, the Oregon Federation for Nursing set as one of its goals the control of the patient-staff ratio. The 1986 contract contained a clause setting up a committee on patient-staff ratios. Under the 1988 contract, a committee of both staff nurses and management nurses established an acuity tool that is included in the present nursing contract (Bill Ganschow, executive vice president OFN 1986–1987, private interview, Seattle, Washington, January, 1991). In Canada, the Manitoba Organization of Nurses Association (union) and the Manitoba Association of Registered Nurses (professional association) allied to support increased government funding for nursing education (Gilchrist, 1987). As the above examples show, not only do actions of unions provide progressive models, but alliances between professional organizations can increase the power of nursing.

In contrast to the strategy by nurses of color and union nurses in forming alliances, white middle-class nursing leaders severed their ties with women's groups and allied themselves with professional groups. At the end of the nineteenth century, nursing groups and women's philanthropic groups were allied around sanitary and hygiene concerns, but by the 1920s nursing identified with professional groups rather than with the concerns of women's groups (Armeny, 1983). In fact, early leaders of nursing rejected identifying with women's concerns. In 1908, for example, the American Nurses' Association (ANA) rejected a resolution supporting women's right to vote, only changing their position to the affirmative in 1915, just five years before the passage of the Nineteenth Amendment (Christy, 1971). ANA's record in support of the Equal Rights Amendment (ERA) is worse, with ANA only coming to support the amendment in 1971. It was not until 1978 that the ANA gave its support to the economic boycott of states that had not ratified the ERA. As of 1982, the National League for Nursing had still not publicly supported the ERA (Heide, 1982). White nursing leaders, in attempting to ignore the reality of sexism, also attempted to follow the professional model of the dominant culture, while black and union nurses recognized the racism and classism in the society. As a result, black nurses allied with other black emancipatory groups. Union nurses have agitated to correct imbalances in pay, hours, and benefits. The latter two groups have not copied the techniques of white male middle-class medicine and as a result are models of empowerment.

ALTERNATIVE FRAMEWORK

Nursing can be categorized as a working-class profession affected by its female heritage. The terms *working class* and *profession* are utilized in order to create and to explore the tension between the two ideas. Acknowledging nursing's female heritage necessitates a gender analysis. By exploring the contrast between the accepted ideas of working-class and professional concerns and by exploring the effects of sexism on nursing, an alternative gendered model for nursing can be formulated.

Inherent in the idea of the working class is the lack of autonomy over use of its skills and reimbursement for its work. Also inherent in the idea of the working class is its supposed connection to people's concrete conditions. Salaries, hours, benefits, and job assignments are subjects that rise here. Nurses do not have control over hours, rate of pay, how many patients they see, what kind of treatment they provide, or the cost of their skill (Allen, 1987). These are priority issues for working nurses. These concrete concerns of nurses, however, do not exclude concerns that have been traditionally relegated to the realm of the "professional."

In defining the notion of profession, the idea of a person's investment in an occupation is assumed. Goals of autonomy, control over education, control over scope of practice, pride in practice, and accountability are the accepted traditional elements of professionals. Nursing, in setting standards for educational requirements and for nursing practice as well as formulating and acting on a code of ethics (Yarling & McElmurry, 1986), displays the desire to place these concerns as priorities along with labor issues.

In juxtaposing the term *working class* with *profession* and owning its female grounding, the biases in the male model of professionalism are eliminated. If class bias is removed, a profession can be considered the same as an occupation, and professionalism a movement that encourages unity. The values of the working-class connection to the concrete realities of the world combined with an altruistic model of professionalism eliminate the hidden exclusionary tactics of the dominant culture model. Nursing, by adopting the term *working-class profession with a female heritage* would be acknowledging both the reality of its working world and its commitment to nursing practice.

CONCLUSION

The rejection of emancipatory, feminist, class, and racial analysis led early nursing leaders to attempt to ally with professional groups rather than women's groups (Armeny, 1983). In attempting to ally with professional groups who achieved status on the basis of exclusion rather than empowerment, nursing lost perspectives from working-class nurses and nurses of color. Emancipatory alliances that black nurses retained were not adopted by white nurses. Instead of utilizing the strengths available from unionism or antiracism, nursing is still weakened by divisions between working-class and management nurses. Retaining the class and racial bias in the dominant culture's model of professionalism has led to a lack of respect for each other as nurses with multiple experiences, skills, and differing learning styles as well as differing experiences of struggle.

DISCUSSION QUESTIONS

1. What are the disadvantages for nursing of following medicine's professionalist model?
2. What are some features of what O'Neill calls "progressive models" for advancing the interests of nurses?
3. Design a public policy initiative that would reflect the possibilities of a "working class profession affected by its female heritage." Explain how it is different from an initiative based on the more narrow, race- and class-bound model of professionalism criticized by O'Neill.
4. O'Neill proposes a postmodern or deconstructionist approach to analyzing professionalism in nursing. In what ways does her approach integrate the postmodern concerns addressed in the chapters by Thompson or Maeda Allman? What elements of a more traditional approach can be found in her analysis?
5. O'Neill sketches an "explanation" of nursing's drive for professionalism. What dimensions of "unacknowledged conditions," "action,"

and "unintended consequences" are included in her explanation (see the discussion of Giddens by Allen)? Are there dimensions she has omitted that you think are important?

REFERENCES

Allen, D. (1987). Professionalism, occupational segregation by gender and control of nursing. *Women & Politics*, 6(3), 1–24.

Armeny, S. (1983). Organized nurses, women philanthropists, and the intellectual bases for cooperation among women, 1918–1920. In E. C. Lagemann (Ed.), *Nursing history: New perspectives, new possibilities* (pp. 13–45). New York: Teachers College Press.

Balser, D. (1987). *Sisterhood & solidarity: Feminism & labor in modern times.* Boston: South End Press.

Baly, M. E. (1987). The Nightingale nurses: The myth and the reality. In C. Maggs (Ed.), *Nursing history: The state of the art* (pp. 33–59). Wolfeboro, NH: Croom Helm.

Baumgart, A. J. (1983). The conflicting demands of professionalism and unionism. *International Nursing Review*, 30(5), 150–155.

Carnegie, M. E. (1986). *The path we tread: Blacks in nursing, 1854–1984.* Philadelphia: J. B. Lippincott.

Christy, T. (1971). Equal rights for women: Voices from the past. *American Journal of Nursing*, 71(2), 288–293.

Davis, A. Y. (1981). *Women, race, and class.* New York: Vintage Books.

Ehrenreich, B. (1975). Health care industry: A theory of industrial medicine. *Social Policy*, 6(3), 4–11.

Ehrenreich, B. (1989). *Fear of falling: The inner life of the middle class.* New York: Harper Perennial.

Ehrenreich, B., & English, D. (1973). *Witches, midwives, and nurses: A history of women healers.* New York: The Feminist Press.

Friedman, A. (1987). Midwifery: Legal or Illegal? A case study of an accused, 1905. In C. Maggs (Ed.), *Nursing history: The state of the art* (pp. 74–87). Wolfeboro, NH: Croom Helm.

Giddings, P. (1984). *When and where I enter: The impact of Black women on race and sex in America.* New York: Bantam Books.

Gilchrist, J. M. (1987). Unionism and professionalism in nursing. *The Canadian Nurse*, 83(10), 31–33.

Heide, W. S. (1982). Feminist activism in nursing and health care. In J. Muff (Ed.), *Socialization, sexism, and stereotyping: Women's issues in nursing* (pp. 255–272). Prospect Heights, IL: Waveland Press.

Hine, D. C. (Ed.). (1985). *Black women in nursing: A documentary history*. New York & London: Garland Publishing.

Hine, D. C. (1989). *Black women in white: Racial conflict and cooperation in the nursing profession: 1890–1950*. Bloomington & Indianapolis: Indiana University Press.

hooks, b. (1984). *Feminist theory: From margin to center*. Boston: South End Press.

Krampitz, S. (1985). The Yale experiment: Innovation in nursing education. In C. Maggs, (Ed.), *Nursing history: The state of the art* (pp. 60–73). Wolfeboro, NH: Croom Helm.

Krampitz, S. (1987). Nursing power, nursing politics. In C. Maggs (Ed.), *Nursing history: The state of the art* (pp. 88–106). Wolfeboro, NH: Croom Helm.

Le Guin, U. (1989). A left-handed commencement address. *Dancing at the edge of the world: Thoughts on words, women, places*. New York: Harper & Row.

Melosh, B. (1982). *"The physician's hand": Work culture in American nursing*. Philadelphia: Temple University Press.

Muff, J. (1982). Why doesn't a smart girl like you go to medical school? The women's movement takes a slap at nursing. In J. Muff (Ed.), *Socialization, sexism, and stereotyping: Women's issues in nursing* (pp. 178–185). Prospect Heights, IL: Waveland Press.

Nutting, M. A., & Dock, L. (1907). *A history of nursing: The evolution of nursing systems from the earliest times to the foundation of the first English and American training schools for nurses Vol. II*. New York & London: G. P. Putnam's Sons/The Knickerbocker Press.

Reverby, S. M. (1987). *Ordered to care: The dilemma of American nursing, 1850–1945*. Cambridge: Cambridge University Press.

Staupers, M. K. (1951). Story of the National Association of Colored Graduate Nurses. In D. C. Hine (Ed.) (1985), *Black women in nursing: A documentary history*. New York & London: Garland Publishing.

Woods, C. Q. (1987). From individual dedication to social activism: Historical development of nursing professionalism. In C. Maggs (Ed.), *Nursing history: The state of the art* (pp. 153–175). Wolfeboro, NH: Croom Helm.

Woods, N. (1981). Women as health care providers. In C. I. Fogel &. N. Woods (Eds.), *Health care of women: A nursing perspective* (pp. 27–39). St. Louis: C. V. Mosby.

Yarling, R. R., & McElmurry, B. J. (1986). The moral foundation of nursing. *Advances in Nursing Science, 8*(2), 63–73.

11

A Critical Analysis of Professionalism in Nursing

Beatrice B. Turkoski

Our understanding of life has been underdeveloped and distorted because our explanations were created by only one half of human kind (Miller, 1989).

INTRODUCTION

As stimulating and invigorating as the present theme is—"Critical Theory—Feminist Theory and Nursing Inquiry"—it is also just a bit frightening. We are talking about revolution here, not of violence, but of a more lasting revolution of social thought. We are, as Moccia (1989) suggests, trying to "find our way out of the chaos into which we have been led by generations of educated men" rather than continuing to be led by non-nurses, accepting the ideologies and paradigms of others, and working within the political and social limits laid down by others. In effect, we are seeking the strength that will allow nursing to grasp an unprecedented opportunity to take the lead in defining a humanistically centered approach to health.

However, the changes that we envision could be purely illusionary and transitory if we fail to understand how the ideas that we want to change were made plausible in nursing history. According to Popkewitz (in press), we need "to look at the ideas of progress and change without being mesmerized by the illusions of change inherent in the rationalization of that progress." The study that I will discuss here (Turkoski, 1989) illustrates how the application of critical and feminist theory strips away illusion and facilitates an emancipated understanding of nursing history and the impact of professionalism in that history.

Professionalism has been a problematic focus of attention for nursing for much of this century. It has often been an area of conflict within nursing and between nursing and forces external to nursing, that is, those forces that seek to control the development of nursing knowledge and those forces that profit from nursing labor. Since the 1960s, as well, with the move to restrict the title *professional* to nurses with academic degrees, the internal rhetoric of professionalism has become increasingly strident and divisive. This move is seen as an effort to establish hierarchies of nursing labor, and to disenfranchise large groups of nurses as "less than professional." The divisiveness and fractionalism within the community of nursing provides yet another opportunity for external forces to control nursing knowledge and practice. Within nursing, the lack of unity also reduces the impact that nursing could have in directing the focus of health care from the current biomedical profit-motivated system to a more humanistically centered and socially responsible model.

Throughout the history of nursing, one paradigm of professionalism has been used as a guide. This traditional [sic] model is defined by predominantly male occupations that claim professional status and the right to determine which occupations shall be deemed professions. This model is also based on a concept that appeals to consistent and universal properties—isolated, free of context, with a neutral "fixed" meaning.

Such an approach to professionalism, without recourse to the conditions from which it arose, the conditions it creates, or the historical discourse which communicates it, has risked miscomprehension of the social, political, and economic realities of professionalism. Thus, nursing has traditionally attempted to measure itself, or has been measured by others, against meanings and definitions of a unilateral world that is based on inherited or adopted concepts and assumed traditions.

Today, after almost a century of destructive controversy and debate, there is a small but increasingly viable expression of skepticism regarding nursing's historically espoused view of professionalism as well as a growing interest in a critical revisionist approach to history and social science per se (Allen, 1987; Freidson, 1970; Larson, 1977; Melosh, 1983; Starr, 1982). This approach suggests that emancipated decision making requires a critical insight into relationships of power; relationships whose strength often lies in their opacity. Thus, this study, developed from a critical philosophy, neither asks traditional questions, nor does it approach professionalism from a trait-set concept.

Rather, this study approaches professionalism as an ideology and incorporates and acknowledges the domination, patriarchy, and asymmetry inherent in traditional professionalism. It illustrates how the acceptance of a particular ideology of professionalism implies an acceptance of a particularized view of knowledge development, ideological purposes, and socialization that serves the dominant social structures. In an effort to more fully understand the relationship between nursing and the ideology of professionalism over time, I ask: "How did the ideology of professionalism appear and change over time in nursing discourse?" and "How does the discourse of nursing professionalism give meaning to changing and competing social structures?" I seek thereby to understand the philosophical origins, constructs, characteristics, and purposes of the ideology of professionalism in nursing.

EXAMINING PROFESSIONALISM AS AN IDEOLOGY

Before discussing the historical implications of the ideology of professionalism in nursing, I will briefly describe the supporting theories, design, and process of the study.

This study is grounded in an intellectual philosophy of "critique" that seeks to understand the relationship between human knowledge and the conditions that produce that knowledge (Geuss, 1981). This approach to developing knowledge implies a view of humankind as capable of determining its own destiny; this is a view of the world as multidimensional, rather than unidimensional (Thompson, 1981). It is a study of changes over time, a resistance to freezing interactive dynamics into one reified view of a special subject, increasing awareness of coercion, frustration, and inequalities of power that lead to domination.

The study is informed by John Thompson's (1984) critical definition of ideology as:

> The image which a social group gives of itself, to itself as a community with a history and an identity . . . a code of interpretation that justifies its own authority . . . that justifies class domination by virtue of distortion . . . that

inverts the order of reality and ideas, and conceals certain features of the social world.

In addition, the feminist philosophy of Eisenstein (1977) is incorporated in this examination of nursing professionalism. The social patriarchy as genderized domination and subjugation is addressed as one component of professional asymmetry.

Thompson's approach to the critical analyses of ideology guided the study design, which is based on the Habermasian (1981) argument that language is the "essential medium" of ideology. In this regard, only through a critical examination of human communications and the actions that relate to those communications will we uncover the distortions and domination in society.

Analysis was directed at actually occurring instances of discourse found in the *American Journal of Nursing* (AJN) between the years 1900 and 1985. This journal was chosen because it is the one nursing publication that has been continuously owned and edited by nurses since 1900, and because it is the sole organ of the major national nursing organizations. As the "voice of nursing," the voice of influence and leadership, the journal "serve(s) as a permanent record of professional progress," and imparts "much valuable information" to the public.

All articles referenced under the index heading "professional" or including "professional" in the title were identified. These articles were then submitted to several careful readings and rigorous notetaking to identify themes and patterns that were then pursued in additional articles. Analysis focused on extended sequences of expression rather than individual semantic units, addressed the themes and attributional associations of professionalism found in the discourse, and identified the ways that the discourse gives meaning to changing and competing social structures. It was designed to examine how ideology incorporates dissimulation, reification, materialism, and patriarchy in such a way as to distort reality so that it appears as "normal" and "natural."

To address the theoretical approaches of this study in a two-dimensional, "fixed" model misses the multidimensional sense of sociohistorical interactions over time. However, the model that follows attempts to incorporate a broad sense of direction for spatially oriented persons. The model attempts to depict how ideology, operating in the medium of language that reifies, dissimulates, and legitimates asymmetry and domination, contributes to an inverted, distorted worldview that neutralizes that same asymmetry and domination.

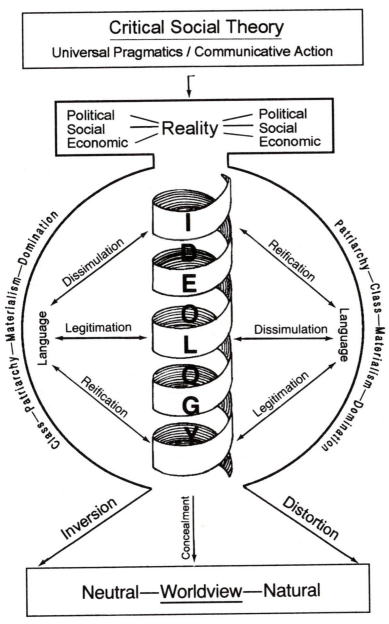

Figure 1
Conceptual Model

THE DISCOURSE OF PROFESSIONALISM IN NURSING

With this brief introduction as background, and assuming that the reading audience has some view of American nursing, let us now examine the relationship between nursing and professionalism that emerged from the present analysis.

Essentially, the discourse surrounding nursing professionalism does support the critical approach to professionalism as an ideology. For nursing, professionalism has been far more than a lattice of ideas, more than a concept, and more than a label. It is, in fact, an image that nursing adopts from prevailing social mores, alters to fit its own situations, and gives of itself to itself and to the community.

It is apparent from the analyses of these eight decades of articles that two primary assumptions were introduced in the early 1900s and perpetuated up till the present: first, that professions hold a social position superior to that of nonprofessions and, second, that being recognized as a profession is a desirable goal for nursing. Rising from this goal, the discourse focuses on legitimating nursing's claim to professional status and on rationalizing action that is viewed as supportive to that claim.

It is further obvious, when evaluating the picture that nursing creates of its own professionalism, that the language distorts and conceals the reality of patriarchy and materialism both in society and in the health care industry. It perpetuates asymmetrical structures of domination between men and women, and between women of different social groups—reinforcing thereby political, and economic power structures external to nursing.

The themes associated with nursing professionalism are highly interrelated and enter virtually every aspect of nursing development. My attempt to separate or "tease out" these areas should be viewed as an arbitrary separation done in the best interests of presenting the material in a coherent manner. Moreover, each of the identified themes should be explored in depth. However, even my brief look at several such themes will illustrate the validity of using a critical approach to sociohistorical research as a means of developing informed understanding.

The Language of Hierarchy and Status

The primary observation gained from my analyses of AJN articles of concern is that nursing has totally and irrevocably adopted and incorporated the prevailing ideas of a social hierarchy predicated on occupation, that is, that professions are at the very peak of an arbitrary designation of social stratification and hierarchy. (It must be noted here that this sense of professionalism is an Anglo-Saxon, predominantly American, concept that developed over time and took on an unchallenged—until recently—neutral and natural appearance during the nineteenth century.)

Throughout the eight decades of nursing discourse, professionalism is referred to as "rank," "an elevated position," a symbol of "social status" that is normally and naturally higher than that accorded to "mere trades," "commerce," or "manual labor." This ingrained idea of professions as occupations of status and rank is illustrated across the decades in assertions that nursing is "more than a calling" and not to be considered "only a trade." It is found in calls for action such as standardizing educational requirements and membership in the national nursing organization that would "raise," elevate," and "bring" nursing to the "divine status of a profession" (notice the word *divine*.) And, it is found in arguments against any action that would be viewed as a threat to nursing's status as a profession, such as chewing gum, wearing the professional uniform and cap in public, participating in labor activities that were "commercial" and "non-professional" because professional nurses "were more interested in service, than in remuneration," or accepting government funding earmarked for "technical and industrial" schools because "nursing by its very tradition belongs with professions rather than trades" and accepting such funds "would raise questions about nursing ever attaining the standing of a profession."

A second hierarchy is also apparent in nursing discourse, a hierarchy among those occupations labeled as professions. Medicine and law (essentially white, Christian, male occupations) are described as the models of "established," "full," "real," and "mature professions." Nursing (essentially a white, Christian, female occupation) is described as a "new," "novice," or "sub-profession." However, in 1900, the readers were assured, and have been continuously assured across the years, that nursing could "move towards a more genuine professional basis," "evolve towards an equal professional standing," "attain full professional status," or "achieve a true professional standing" only by emulating the "true" or "model" professions.

On the one hand, the adoption of this arbitrary social hierarchy, as mentioned, appeared to legitimate asymmetrical power structures between nurses and clients—incorporating a sense of elitism within the very work of nursing. On the other hand, the acceptance and integration within nursing of this model of social class hierarchy served to perpetuate a system in which women, and nurses as women, were occupationally and socially dominated and subjugated. Additionally, the discourse suggested that it was desirable for nursing to follow the examples of "model" professions so that nursing could eventually reach the "promised land" of "full" professionalism. Attaining "full" professionalism would thus legitimate as normal or natural those nursing actions which perpetuate asymmetrical power relationships between various "classes" of women who went into nursing.

For nursing, the themes related to the adopted elite view of professionalism are essentially two-directional. In one direction the discourse argues that nursing is entitled to professional status because it has met certain arbitrary requirements. In the other direction, the discourse argues that nursing must redouble its efforts to meet certain requirements in order to achieve "full" acceptance as a profession. In the following discussion of the analyses, I will attempt to illustrate aspects of this two-directional discourse.

Professionalism as Market Protection

One particular theme related to nursing professionalism is that of market protection.

Early authors stressed that recognition and acceptance of "organized" (membership in the national/state organization), "trained" (graduating from a recognized training school) nurses as professionals would protect "those deserving trained young women from the predators, those washerwomen masquerading in white." In later years, private duty registries, registration, and mandatory licensing were directly related to protecting the market for "professional nurses" from the "make-believe nurses" and those untrained "non-professionals" serving as nurses. In more recent times, the same market protection relationship with professionalism can be found in the movements for "entry into practice" and advanced certification.

Although this idea of market protection was (and still is) posited as a strong argument for those actions that were supposedly related to maintaining or achieving professional rank, it also perpetuated a distinct classism and asymmetrical hierarchy within nursing based on assumptions of asymmetrical "worth" among nursing activities. By defining professional as based on an academic education, women from lower economic classes and minorities were excluded from the rank of professional.

Moreover, via critical philosophy and the contrasting of the discourse of professionalism with the realities of political and economic markets, it becomes clear that the ideology of professionalism distorted reality. For, in truth, nursing has never been protected in the marketplace. In the first two or three decades of this century, for example, hospitals were almost completely staffed with free student labor. Graduated, trained, or professional nurses (the terms were for many years used interchangeably) were dumped out into the community following their student years to find employment in private practice. The general public had little knowledge or interest in whether their nurses were "professionals." Moreover, since it was "blatantly unprofessional" to advertise, these professional nurses had to rely on pharmacists, physicians, or the established hospital registries for referrals. Such agencies could then mandate wages, schedules, dress, and behavior.

Later in the century, market protectionism proved effective, as exclusionary hospital regulations appeared to support hierarchical divisions among nursing labor. However, one must consider that most regulation and legislation was reactive rather than proactive, and most of it was restrictive to nursing, rather than expansive. Moreover, the men who controlled the economic and political arenas of health care could, and still can, change or subvert the intent of these laws to support their particular agendas—witness the recent RTC* debacle.

Altruism and Service—The Devaluing of Nursing Labor

The two-directional aspects of professionalism are also found in the language that associates professionalism with altruism and service, language that clearly placed nursing in a subservient position in the health care arena.

In nursing discourse, altruism and service become a form of self-coercion that makes economic inequality and asymmetry appear normal, natural, and even desired as a badge of professional status. Nursing is entitled to the status of a profession, authors argued (and many still do), because "nursing is a calling" and "is more interested in service to mankind" than nonprofessions, and because nurses do not "work primarily for pecuniary gain" but "have a sense of noblesse oblige as a guiding principle." Professional nurses, it was thus argued, differ from "non-professionals" with "purely commercial interests" because professional nurses are, in fact, "non-commercial" and "without interest in financial gain or economic equality."

Graduated nurses, employed in private practice and most often treated as, and paid less than, servants or those washer women from whom their professionalism was supposed to protect them, were exhorted to maintain their fees at minimal levels, not to better serve the needy, but to maintain the "non-

---

*RTC refers to the recent attempt by the American Medical Association to introduce a new level of institutional employees, trained for less than a year, who would assume nursing responsibilities.

commercial" aspect of their professionalism. Those who sought to increase their fees were described as "non-professional" and "commercial," and their commercialism was not only described as "un-professional," but they were considered a "danger" to the professional standing of other nurses in the community.

This same sense of altruism and service also incorporated the social standing of women and women's labor within the context of nursing professionalism. Readers of the *American Journal of Nursing* were advised that even though they were professionals, nurses were all women and, as women, they should "never expect the same wage scale as men"—"after all," it was stated, "the service of nursing was more important than the remuneration."

During the depression of the 1930s, major social changes appeared to force nurses from their relative autonomy in private practice into the servitude of hospital institutions. First, the depression meant that there were very few private citizens who could afford the care of a nurse; thus, there were many hundreds of nurses without income. Second, the federal government began to support the health care industry, and increasing numbers of citizens began to use hospitals, creating increased demand for nursing labor. At the same time, with other occupational avenues opening for women, fewer students were recruited to fill the need for hospital labor. As a result, hospitals began to employ graduate (registered, professional) nurses—at wages determined as the amount that hospitals expended for housing and feeding students. Thus, nurses forever exchanged the relative autonomy of private practice for the servitude (and very tenuous security) of institutional employment at wages set by these institutions. This very act was a major move from the societal consensus of a profession—the men in the "true" "model" professions of medicine or law that nursing sought somehow to emulate did not work as employees of institutions, nor were their economic rewards determined by any external body beyond that of the prevailing market for their services.

In this changing institutional setting, the same kind of convoluted association of altruism and service with professionalism was used to rationalize, normalize, and distort subjugation and domination in any relationship between nursing labor and the hospital industry. When nurses sought economic rewards similar to other employees, they were (and are) consistently cautioned by nursing leaders not to request increased wages from "hard-pressed hospitals." The reasons here are as insidious as they are effective: first, as professionals, nurses must consider that "the cause of the institution comes first," and second, since nursing's claim to professional status is so tenuous, "we [nurses] must make sacrifices, lest we lose the priceless position that we have gained."

This distortion and dissimulation of reality has plagued nursing ever since. Placing the commercial, capital interests of hospitals above their own need for economic remuneration as a measure of accepting "professional" status devalued nursing labor in relation to other hospital employees. (Here I would urge you to consider how stridently these same arguments, first heard several decades ago, are again presented in nursing discourse today.)

When labor unions began actively seeking to recruit nurses, the employed nurses were cautioned by nursing leaders (writing in the *American Journal of Nursing*) that belonging to any labor organization with purely "commercial" interests was "blatantly unprofessional." In fact, any labor action against the institutions, it was asserted, was "un-professional" and would place nursing in the same category as trades or specifically industrial occupations.

Eventually, when the national nurses' organization succumbed to internal pressures from constantly deteriorating nurse-hospital relations, it was argued that as "true professionals" nurses did not join "outside" labor organizations; rather, they should use their professional organization for any labor negotiations. This idea infects the language of professionalism with a troubling dichotomy. It suggested that nurses should rely on the same organization that had for decades advocated actions grounded in a view of professionalism that devalued nursing and nursing labor to arbitrate with the very power structures from which nursing wanted recognition of its professional status.

To an institution, the consistent and pervasive association of professionalism with altruism and service not only affected direct employment relationships, but also the development of nursing education. Operating from the conviction that "real" professions solved the question of supply and demand within the context of the profession, nursing has followed an erratic, seesaw approach to supplying inexpensive nursing labor for the hospital industry by manipulating educational requirements. When there was an abundance of nursing labor, moves toward increasing requirements for training were identified as "long overdue developments in the progress of nursing toward full professionalism." When there were acute shortages of nursing labor, restrictive requirements were abandoned and vigorous recruiting campaigns reinforced the idea of student labor as "learning a profession" and "providing a service."

This very argument also precluded nursing's move from institutional training to academic education. During the early 1900s, when the idea of moving nursing education to academic campuses first surfaced, a primary argument against such a move was that hospitals could not function without free nursing labor—of course they couldn't; they might have had to actually pay for that labor. However, the nursing discourse of professionalism argued that it was a professional responsibility of nursing to maintain the supply of labor for the hospitals, and any move toward academic education must be so designed as to continue the provision of student labor.

In the mid 1950s, this same argument became the basis for the design of two-year nursing programs. The two-year concept, however, was a reactive response to a demand for increased quantity, not quality, of nursing labor. Thus, in the language of professionalism, the argument that a "true" profession solves supply and demand problems from within concretized a societal image of nursing—a nurse is a nurse is a nurse. It is not hard to see that, just as the goals of economic equality were subverted to the goals of professionalism, so were the goals of education of lesser import than professionalism.

Dress as a Symbol of Professionalism

Another theme that illustrates how nursing altered the prevailing concept of professionalism can be found in the language that overtly associates particular dress requirements—the "holy uniform"—with professionalism. The discourse that addresses the symbols of uniform, cap, and pin as a "sign of professionalism" is consistent across the years. The cap is described as a symbol of "purity" and "virtue" (in order to be accepted for professional nurses' training, young women had to present written testimonials as to their purity) or as a symbol of "calling" (both the cap and the language are highly reminiscent of Christian religious orders in which women were certainly as dominated and subjugated by institutionalized patriarchy as were nurses).

The white of the graduate's uniform (students were clothed in dark-colored uniforms—a highly symbolic manifestation of an internal hierarchy) is described as a symbol of professional "status," and readers were cautioned about the "unprofessional" aspect of wearing this symbol "of their professional rank" on public streets or streetcars. (As an aside, chewing gum, loud voices, and hilarity were also "unprofessional"—according to the discourse of professionalism). Later, when beauticians, stewardesses, and people of "lesser status" had the gall to appear in white uniformesque clothing, the outrage in the language of nurses was almost palpable.

This relationship of dress and professionalism reveals how the actual language may change but the internalized concept does not. During the last few decades, when students and practicing nurses have consistently fought against the imposed institutional regimentation of uniforms and caps, they have argued from the point that "true professionals" do not wear uniforms. Their argument that questions the relationship between a particular style of wearing apparel and the ability to think or apply that thought appears to challenge one distortion in the nursing ideology of professionalism. However, their argument is also predicated on the integration of professional status and rank, as they point out that "true," "real," and "accepted" professionals do not wear uniforms—only nonprofessionals wear uniforms.

Classism, Genderism, and Racism in Nursing Professionalism

The asymmetrical concepts of status and rank associated with nursing professionalism also extended to classism, genderism, and racism in ways that make these social asymmetries appear as normal and natural parts of society. Beginning with the first issue of the *American Journal of Nursing*, the victorian ideals of womanly submissiveness, duty, and servitude were virtually concretized in the basic idea of nursing professionalism. Even after the horrors of World War II, in the late 1940s, this ideal way was still found in relationship to the word *professional*.

Thus, we find descriptions of the professional nurses as "women of quality, sensible, kindly, home-makers, endowed with sympathy, brains, and tact." Professional nurses were described as "gentlewomen," "women of culture," "noble with non-commercial motives," "dutiful and self-sacrificing." This idea of womanly character was, in essence, an upper-class distinction that reflects the backgrounds of the early leaders in nursing—mainly women from upper-class homes, better educated than 90 percent of the women in that era, and brought up in a time when the epitome of upper-class womanliness was "service."

By the middle of the first decade of the century however, the wellspring of women of means who were willing to accept the unbelievably hard task of nursing as a "calling" grew smaller. Yet, the need for more nurses in the almshouses and hellholes that passed for hospitals was increasing. As a result, nurses' training, the opportunity to become a "professional," follow a "calling," and at the same time learn a skill that they could eventually use in private practice (remember, ordinary people who underwent surgery, gave birth, and died were nursed through their illnesses at home) was used to recruit women from the middle classes to staff those hospitals. Professionalism became a banner for recruitment to schools of nursing. This call or promise of achieving social status through professionalism was extremely effective at a time in history when women did not leave home to work at "regular" jobs and did not live alone without chaperons. Women were socially viewed as immoral temptresses, their brains were perceived as smaller than men's, they were reported to be too ignorant to vote, and, of course, they could not own property. Thus nursing, presented as a form of social status and rank, could be considered to provide a sense of self through the process of professionalization.

However, the educational requirements for entry into "professional" nursing did, and still do, discriminate against women of color and women from the lower economic classes. Seldom did these women have the opportunity to meet the educational admission requirements, and seldom could they afford the time required for professional nurses' training—and much of the same holds true today.

Within the ideological discourse of professionalism, one finds, during the first half of this century, the idea that women of lower classes could find their place in practical nursing. Then, in the 1950s, the introduction of two-year programs of nursing education was designed to recruit women from the lower economic levels and minorities. As we all know, these nurses took the same credentialing exams as graduates from hospital training programs and academic programs, and thus were essentially entitled to the rank of professional by virtue of their status as registered or licensed nurses. In the 1960s, the movement to label these nurses as *technical* (hospital nursing programs were dying out) and those educated in academia as *professional* was viewed as a form of asymmetrical division, an enforced, hierarchical disenfranchisement for *technical* nurses—thus perpetuating an internal classism within the ideology of professionalism.

Professional nursing, the act of nursing, has also been described in purely genderized terms as: "women's mission, ministry, humanitarian service," a "service of womanly duty and conscience," "the noblest and most womanly of professions," which involves womanly virtues in "faithful, intelligent, obedient, humble service to the general public." Such descriptions of nursing as a profession specifically involved in "women's work" reinforced the assumption that nursing practice is essentially related to one biological makeup. Thus, the sex-segregated social order of society was perpetuated in nursing's ideology of professionalism. Is it any wonder, then, that we have few men in nursing? Even as late as 1970, seven out of ten *American Journal of Nursing* articles that included references to nurses as professionals referred to them as "she's"? And those that did refer to males in nursing used "men nurses"—something like "women doctors," don't you think?

Racism was also internalized in the professional ideology of nursing. Nursing adopted the discriminatory practices of racism not only in their all white schools and hospitals, but in the national organization of professional nurses. Even as late as 1956, when discussing segregation practices in state organizations, the voice of nursing leadership argued that this was not a professional concern, that taking a professional stand was not within the interests of the national organization, and suggested that individual members of the profession make personal decisions about integration.

An Elite View of Political Activism

One would think, after examining the picture that nursing painted of itself as a profession, that the women who wanted status, rank, and position would have then supported the various women's movements for emancipation and suffrage. But they did not! In the years following 1909, when the "women's movement" agitated for emancipitation and suffrage, professional nurses were cautioned that the only legitimate political interests of nursing were those directly concerned with the problems of health care. Fifty years later the same silence surrounded the movement for the Equal Rights Amendment (ERA). Only in 1971, did the "official," professional voice of nursing finally endorse the ERA.

Across the decades, nurses were continually cautioned that correct "professional" activity was concerned with health-related activities, not political activism. Thus, we find in the picture of nursing professionalism a certain support for legislation addressing general health needs, but very little commitment to changing the conditions that aggravated those needs. Obviously, the proscribed, elite view of professionalism was to take the "safe" route, supporting only those concerns considered as such: reactive in every essence, rather than proactive in any instance. This observation does not preclude the political involvement of individual nurses or mean that certain groups of nurses were not involved in effecting social change—many were. The issue here is what the "official voice of nursing" identified as legitimate "professional" action.

CONCLUSION

In this study, I did not answer the eternal questions: "Is nursing a profession?" or "Which nurse is professional?" I did not intend to. The significance of my approach to nursing professionalism as ideology is this: it adds to the understanding of how assumptions and implications of an ideology adopted from a patriarchal, positivistic view have contributed to the current condition in nursing. It illustrates how decisions were made plausible through language used as a means of distortion and concealment. It identifies how, through the decades, the themes that nursing associated with professionalism had altered meanings which incorporated a subjugated position of women and women's work in both the occupation and social arenas, while maintaining a facade, an illusion, that these conditions were neutral and natural. And further, it identifies how a commitment to the ideology of professionalism has focused on power strategies that seem incompatible with the nursing ethic of caring—elitism, disenfranchisement, subordination, classism, racism, and genderism, as well as destructive approaches to service and altruism.

A study such as this, from a philosophy of critique, has implications for further research in nursing and feminism. Knowledge developed within the framework of critical social theories can be enlightening and emancipating. Only by identifying and understanding how political, social, and economic domination and asymmetry is rationalized and legitimated through language can we demystify the constraints and coercion in health care and self-consciously frame equitable relationships within nursing and between nursing and society.

DISCUSSION QUESTIONS

1. Turkoski develops her critique of professionalist discourse in hopes of facilitating a move by nursing toward a "humanistically centered approach to health." What features of professionalist discourse does she see as incompatible with this approach to health care?

2: How have the attributes of professionalism changed during the 80 years analyzed by Turkoski?

3. Turkoski, like Allen and other authors in this collection, focuses not on "professionalism," but on the "discourse of professionalism." What is the difference and what advantages does a discourse analysis have for nurses within critical and feminist traditions? Why was her study not directed toward "Is nursing a profession" or "Which nurse is professional?"

4. Discuss how you might approach the advancement of nursing as an occupation without incorporating the aspects of professionalism criticized by Turkoski?

REFERENCES

[There are more than 100 brief quotes from the eight decades of the *American Journal of Nursing*—neither time nor space would permit identifying each and every one—however all *American Journal of Nursing* reference citations are available from the author.]

Allen, D. (1987). Professionalism, occupational segregation by gender and control of nursing. *Women in Politics, 7*, 1–24.

Eisenstein, Z. (1977). Constructing a theory of capitalist patriarchy and the 'case for socialist feminism. *The Insurgent Sociologist, 7*(3), 2–18.

Freidson, R. (1970). *Professional dominance: The structure of medical care.* Chicago: Aldine-Atherton.

Geuss, R. (1981). *The idea of a critical theory: Habermas and the Franfurt school.* Cambridge: Cambridge University Press.

Habermas, J. (1981). *Theory of communication action* (Vol. 1) (T. McCarthy, Trans., 1984). Boston: Beacon Press.

Larson, M. (1977). *The rise of professionalism.* Berkeley: University of California Press.

Melosh, B. (1983). *The physician's hand; Work, culture and conflict in American nursing.* Philadelphia: Temple University Press.

Miller, J. (1986). *Toward a new psychology of women.* Boston: Beacon Press.

Moccia, P. (1988). Curriculum revolution: An agenda for change. In *Curriculum revolution: Mandate for change.* New York: National League for Nursing.

Popkewitz, T. (in press). History in education science: Educational science as history. In *Educational Enquiry: Approaches to Research.* Geelong, Australia.

Starr, P. (1982). *The social transformation of American medicine.* New York: Basic Books.

Thompson, J. (1981). *Critical hermeneutics: A study in the thought of Paul Ricoeur and Jurgen Habermas.* Cambridge: Cambridge University Press.

Thompson, J. (1984). *Studies in the theory of ideology.* Berkeley: University of California Press.

Turkoski, B. (1989). A critical analysis of the discourse of professionalism in nursing. (Doctoral dissertation, University of Wisconsin, 1989), *Dissertation Abstracts International.*

12

Perceptions and Feelings of Nurses About Horizontal Violence as an Expression of Oppressed Group Behavior

Lois Napier Skillings

*I*ntergroup conflict among nurses is a problem which prevents unity and collective power in nursing. Roberts (1983), for example, has used the concept of horizontal violence as an expression of oppressed group behavior to explain this phenomenon.

In this research, I explored perceptions and feelings of nurses about horizontal violence as an expression of oppressed group behavior. The study consisted of dialogue between six white, female nurses and myself about oppression in nursing generally and how oppression promotes horizontal violence in nursing, specifically in the hospital context. These women work in different hospital settings in Northern New England. Three are staff nurses and three hold nursing management positions. My research was guided by emancipatory, participatory, and feminist research methods.

As a nurse, I believe that issues like horizontal violence, power relations, and domination should be explored. Consciousness raising about horizontal violence can help nurses to critically analyze unequal power relationships within the hierarchy of the health care industry. Dialogue about nurses' relationships with each other may enhance awareness of the reasons for intergroup conflict. In turn, this may lead to increased unity and collective autonomy in nursing. Additionally, this heightened sensitivity to the influence of unequal power relations and domination may positively affect nurses' relationships with patients. Ultimately, perhaps a greater sense of individual self-worth and self-esteem may arise through the experience of empowerment of ourselves and others.

Guiding this study was the naturalistic paradigm of qualitative research. This paradigm emphasizes that research is value-laden and that it is impossible to separate the researcher from the research (Lincoln & Guba, 1985). It is important, therefore, to name myself and my motivation for this exploration and personal experience of consciousness raising throughout the process of this work. I am a married 34-year-old, white, middle-class woman from a working-class family origin. I have a young daughter and two grown stepchildren. I have been a nurse for 13 years. My clinical experience includes medical-surgical and emergency nursing. Additionally, I have been a head nurse and a nursing supervisor and have held a nursing administration position.

When I initially began this work, I feared that the focus on this particular aspect of nurses' relationships may be perceived by some as quite negative. In addition, horizontal violence is not at all the norm of my everyday experience in nursing. I am constantly amazed at other nurses' capacity to love, respect, and support one another, and I feared that focusing on those moments when this does not occur would be negative and destructive. However, since my nursing school days, I have been aware that intergroup conflict exists in nursing. I have watched and felt the pain and frustration that results from negative and destructive behavior. The fragmentation of specialty groups, competition, and rivalry are but a few of the collective expressions of intergroup conflict I have experienced.

Then, six years ago during my first graduate nursing course, I read Marilyn French's (1985) *Beyond Power*. This introduction to feminist theory affected me deeply, and I found that my old way of living in the world began to crumble. As a new way of feminist concerns emerged, I began to question my ability to live comfortably in the world of male-defined reality of hierarchy and domination. I also came to realize that nurses' relationships were influenced by the dynamics of power in the structures in which we work and the world in which we live. From there I began my journey of trying to reconcile the dichotomy separating these two worlds. Above all, my desire to reach an expanded understanding of power and praxis led me to the present research.

LITERATURE REVIEW

Domination and Oppressed Group Behavior

Lorde (1984) argues that "there is no hierarchy of oppressions." To be oppressed is to be "other than." Oppression stems from intolerance of differences, which include age, race, class, ethnic and cultural backgrounds, and gender and sexual orientation. Freire (1970) suggests that those who dominate do so out of self-interest and prescribe and define reality for all in order to serve this interest. The oppressed, who are denied of freedom, self-expression, and self-definition by constraints imposed by others, have been described as exhibiting common reactions to oppressive contexts (Fanon, 1963; Freire, 1970).

Freire (1970) suggests that since reality is defined by the oppressor, the oppressed internalize the consciousness of the oppressor as the "preferable" way of living in the world. This internalization of oppressive values causes the oppressed to deny self and cultural identity. As Fanon (1963) describes them, they become "indistinct masses," lacking identification with their own culture, which they have come to view negatively, yet never truly assimilating into the oppressor's culture because of their "otherness."

According to Freire (1970), the attempt by those oppressed to effect assimilation into the dominant culture causes their marginality. The oppressed find themselves on the margin of one culture, which will never let them in, looking back on another culture, which they have come to view with contempt. In the cultural void of their marginal position, the oppressed seem to adhere to the oppressors with an "insatiable attraction" as they aspire to be like them.

Because of their marginality, the oppressed often exhibit low self-esteem and self-hatred. As a result, members of oppressed groups become fragmented, compartmentalized, and wrought with intergroup conflict. Fanon (1963) described how the oppressed internalize the value of aggression or dominance held by the oppressor and are unable to directly express aggression toward the oppressor because of submissiveness caused by marginality, self-hatred, and low self-esteem. Thus, aggression is expressed horizontally, where it is perceived to be safe to do so, and is an attempt to relieve the tension caused by oppression.

Freire (1970) identified this characteristic of oppressed groups as *horizontal violence*, the means by which oppression is perpetuated. Lacking internal unity and remaining divided, the oppressed do not have the strength to overcome their oppressor (Fanon, 1963). Freire (1970) has further described the characteristics of oppressed groups as cooperative. By perpetuating the status quo, they create barriers to freedom or liberation.

Oppressed Group Behavior in Nursing

Melosh (1982) and Reverby (1989) trace the historical evolution of nursing as a subordinate group within the health care industry and describe how ingrained this definition is in nursing culture and values. Reverby (1987) defines the subordination of nursing by describing the impact of society's devaluing the concept of caring. Lack of autonomy in the work of devalued caring, coupled with the patriarchal structure of the hospital and medicine, combine to create an oppressive reality for nursing. Additionally, Reverby (1989) has described the ethnic, racial, educational, and class differences among nurses as dividing forces, preventing nurses from achieving the solidarity that could come from common gender.

Other researchers have explored the effects of domination on nursing in the literature and described them as contributing to nursing's oppressed group behavior (Ashley, 1980; Chinn and Wheeler, 1985; Keen, 1988; Mullen, 1987; Roberts, 1983). Greenleaf (1982), in particular, has examined the politics of self-esteem in nursing and has argued that nursing's inferior self-definition stems from being defined as inferior by others. This low self-esteem represents an internalization of the values of the dominant culture, the medical and institutional hierarchy, and results in a loss of cultural identity in nursing, self-hatred, and marginal behaviors (Ashley, 1980; Roberts, 1983). Because of this, nurses have been described as a fragmented group with false loyalties and a tendency toward intergroup conflict or horizontal violence.

Ashley (1980) has described horizontal violence in nursing as overt, while Mullen (1987) has focused on its more subtle and symbolic characteristics. Ashley (1973) has also pointed out that horizontal violence in nursing may be abstracted to include the elitism caused by subscribing to a professional ideology that segregates women according to position and educational preparation. Roberts (1983) suggests that marginal leaders within oppressed groups who allow, create, or perpetuate power-over relationships, as evidenced by hierarchy, control, or submission, are demonstrating horizontal violence.

Such marginal behavior by nursing leaders results in continued oppression. As described by Chinn and Wheeler (1985), "traits deriving from a state of oppression and yet viewed as desirable by nurses are even more damaging to the profession, in that they are not recognized as actually perpetuating the oppressing system that the group wishes to overcome" (p. 76).

Critical Social Theory and Feminist Theory

As a paradigm for research, critical social theory defines knowledge development as being directly linked to contextual social and historical realities. Schroyer (1973) argues that "too often the knowledge produced (by contemporary social science) becomes useful only as a means to control 'social problems': and to re-establish a social equilibrium that takes for granted the existing institutional constellation" (p. 25). Critical social theory provides an alternative to this approach of knowledge development.

Critical scholarship has important implications for the study of oppression in nursing. Thompson (1987) defines critical scholarship as "a pattern of thought and action that challenges institutionalized power relations or relations of domination in the social reality of nursing" (p. 28). Allen, Benner, and Diekelmann (1986) argue that critical social science "establish(s) the conditions for open, unconstrained communication," thus promoting free discourse. According to Stevens (1989, p. 67), through a process of conscientization, relations of dominance can be uncovered that can "demystify the ideology that rationalizes unequal power relations."

Feminist theory is a "worldview that values women and confronts systematic injustices based on gender" (Chinn & Wheeler, 1985, p. 74). Feminism critiques the male-defined worldview that, according to French (1985), elevates above all else the acquisition of power and control over nature. The connection between feminism and nursing has been described as imperative as nurses examine both the barriers to care for our patients (MacPherson, 1989a) and our relationships with one another (Chinn & Wheeler, 1985). In this study, I have combined such theories of feminism and critical social science to provide a framework for exploring horizontal violence as a characteristic of oppressed group behavior in nurses.

According to Freire, (1970), the oppressed must perceive the reality of oppression "not as a closed world from which there is no exit, but as a limiting situation which they can transform" (p. 38). This transformation begins with the uncovering of the existence of domination by those who are themselves oppressed (Schroyer, 1973). This research was based on consciousness raising through dialogue with nurses about oppression and how horizontal violence serves to perpetuate it.

RESEARCH QUESTIONS

This study explores the following research questions: What are the perceptions and feelings of hospital nurses concerning horizontal violence? In what circumstances, if any, do they feel violence is expressed?

METHODOLOGY

I conducted the present research as exploratory study designed from a qualitative perspective (described by Lincoln & Guba, 1985) using the axioms of the naturalistic paradigm with a feminist, participatory approach. I further based the study design on Connors (1988), Lather (1986), Maguire (1987), Oakley (1988), and Thompson's (1990) discussion of this same approach.

Feminist participatory research attempts to uncover oppression and express the realities of women via dialogue between the researcher and the participants. Within this nonhierarchical relationship, there is the assumption that the participant has experience and knowledge to share and is capable of critical reflection and analysis (Maguire, 1987).

Lather (1986) has described the consciousness raising which results from participatory research as emancipatory. According to Lather, "the goal of emancipatory research is to encourage self-reflection and deeper understanding on the part of the persons being researched" (p. 266), thus "to empower the oppressed to come to understand and change their own oppressive realities" (p. 260); "It is research as praxis" (p. 258). By connecting this emancipatory approach to critical social theory, Thompson (1990) suggests that "critical researchers are committed to . . . an active, non-elitist engagement with participants to address social injustices" (p. 266).

The present study sample consisted of nurses who practice in the hospital setting as staff nurses or as nurse managers and who have been involved in some experience of feminist consciousness raising. A snowball sample included three staff nurses and three nurses in hospital management positions who were at least minimally aware of the concepts of oppressed group behavior or horizontal violence. The women chose pseudonyms as a way to personalize their stories. Lillian, Margaret, and Maude are staff nurses; Charlotte, Judy, and Julia are in nursing management positions.

The participants are white, middle-class women who range in age from 35 to 45. Their years of experience in nursing range from 8 to 24 years. Their nursing education varies, including diploma, baccalaureate, and master's preparation. The participants work in different settings including small and medium community hospitals and large urban hospital emergency departments, critical-care units, and a medical-surgical unit. The nurses in management positions include one director of nursing, one nurse manager (head nurse), and one assistant head nurse.

Taped, semistructured individual meetings were held with each participant twice between April 1990 and October 1990. Each meeting lasted 60 to 90 minutes. Additionally, a group meeting was held using the feminist process of group interaction described in Wheeler and Chinn's (1984) *Peace and Power*. The meeting was called to allow for "negotiation of meaning" during the data analysis (Lather, 1986; Thompson, 1990) as well as to check for construct validity, face validity, and catalytic validity as described by Lather (1986) and Thompson (1990). Construct validity was described as a process of giving careful attention to guard against imposing ideas on study participants and of showing respect for their unique experiences. I sought construct validity by sharing the data and asking for feedback from participants during the group meeting. I also sought face validity, in which participants and researcher experience mutual recognition as the data emerge.

Another purpose of the group meeting was ensuring catalytic validity, by which the research process and the emerging data move the participants toward a new understanding and opportunity for transformation of their lived experience. The experience of shared consciousness raising in a group setting provided a collective voice with ideas for supporting one another to overcome oppressive realities.

The data were processed according to tasks of unitizing, categorizing, and identifying themes (Lincoln & Guba, 1985). As a result of this analysis, three major themes, or findings, emerged.

FINDINGS

Theme: In nursing, oppression is a reality that is multidimensional and socially constructed.

In the real world, staff nurses know their place. —Julia

In the first theme that emerged from the dialogues, the women described the oppression they experience as a combined result of the organizational environment of the hospital and the relationship between nursing and medicine. They also shared their feelings about how gender relations, class relations, and perceptions of the role of the nurse are mutually reinforcing and serve to perpetuate the nurses' oppression. The following narrative illustrates these many dimensions of oppression in nursing:

> Margaret: *In general, I don't feel that nurses get respect [from physicians]. Male physicians and female physicians do not treat nurses on a peer level or a colleague level, although some of the women physicians will give lip service to that. "Well, we're all women and we're all in this together." But, when it comes right down to brass tacks, they're just as patronizing and demanding . . . [Physicians are] just not respectful of me, of who I am and what I know as a person. We get into quite a few power struggles in the department because of that . . .*

Many dialogues illustrated how gender and class relations contribute simultaneously to feelings of oppression in nursing. Some participants related unequal power relationships between nurses and physicians specifically to class differences. Maude described this tension in the following dialogue:

> Maude: *Well, there is a very definite class issue—it's the people who get their hands dirty versus the people who can stand off and look at what's happening. It's the same flavor that you get when you have a physician who stands back and lets the nurse put the bedpan under the patient that is near his left hand because he does not want to get dirty. It's not his job. It's not his place. He's above that. . . . And that's all also because he has a paper that says he's been to school for years and that gives him the right to move away from the dirty work. Isn't that why everybody becomes a white collar worker? . . .*

Study participants discussed ways in which class relations among nurses contribute to feelings of oppression. Some participants described nursing as a step up the social hierarchy; some described nursing as a step down. Participants also described the institutionalized oppression that they experience by working in the hospital. Julia described her feelings of institutional power relationships in the following dialogue:

> Julia: *I'd like to think that we've made some progress, and I often feel powerful in my position . . . but when I'm forced to look at how much of the bottom line . . . how much influence we really have, [I see] that I really don't have any power.*

Each participant told how oppression is influenced by the society in which we live, the institutions in which we work, and issues such as class distinctions, gender, and our relationships with the dominant culture of medicine

This oppressive reality was also described by the participants as affecting relationships among nurses, which became the second theme of this research.

Theme: As a result of oppression, nurses experience and participate in horizontal violence, and this experience is painful.

> *There is this big they out there in a white uniform that we all get to blame things on*—Lillian

The second theme that emerged from the dialogues was the existence of horizontal violence as an expression of oppressed group behavior in nursing. Some dialogues described how horizontal violence can become the culture of a nursing unit, and how this can negatively affect patient care. Participants spoke of intershift or unit rivalry, competition, and bickering, which is experienced in both overt and subtle ways. They shared their stories about the lack of support they receive from their colleagues when they are different: different in their relationships with patients, different, for example, as a lesbian, and different as an "outsider" or "newcomer." Most participants described how they painfully experienced horizontal violence, as in the following narrative:

> Judy: *The absolute worst that can never be matched again no matter who was on the other side, was a a new grad. I mean, just the absolute worst. You would have thought that there were so many nurses in the world . . . that the whole idea was like a hazing and to just sort of see who you could torture the most and just see how they bore up under the torture. I mean, it seemed just about like that. And there were very many people . . . just trying to catch me . . . I was just aware of it every day that I went to work . . . (They) wanted to sort of fight with me about every little thing. "Oh, you didn't sign off this order" or "Did you do this?"*—*some very little detail about the patient's care.*

For one nurse, horizontal violence included clear examples of sexual assault and harassment that were not confronted by her co-workers and management. Because of the way she was different from the other nurses and her "outsider" status, she experienced the humiliation and pain of sexual harassment without any support from her colleagues:

> Margaret: *When I first came [to the department] . . . what I found was that the men, [specifically] the surgeons and the paramedics, were often very loose with their hands and their hugs . . . I used to walk away and say "please don't do that" and I got no support. I . . . talked to my head nurse about it and she said, "Oh, you're just being a prude." And I talked to the head of the department, who happened to be a woman, who said that she*

would say something about it but nothing ever happened. . . . Other nurses who didn't know me at the time, because I had just started working there, wouldn't defend me either. They just kept saying I was a prude and that [this behavior from these men] was okay. . . . I was down in the lounge one time and a surgeon literally, jokingly according to him, attacked me and laid me down on the couch and got on top of me. There was another nurse in the room and she was laughing and thought it was funny. As people began to know me, it became known that I was a lesbian [about] a year after I'd been there. So now, it was not only that I was a prude, but I was a lesbian. So then I got double whammied . . . they don't understand that this (harassment) is not healthy for me. It's not healthy for them. And, it's very uncomfortable.

In describing their experiences of horizontal violence, the participants acknowledged that the people who were acting this way were doing so out of a sense of powerlessness. Actually, there were discussions about how the idea of horizontal violence can lead to interpretations that blame the victim. Participants felt uncomfortable with victim blaming and did not want to blame nurses for unintended, unconscious actions in oppressive contexts. However, all of the women described the pain or isolation they had experienced as a result of horizontal violence. Three of the participants talked openly about experiences in which they found themselves participating in horizontal violence or times when they felt hostile toward their nursing colleagues.

Some participants discussed the fragmentation they feel exists in nursing as a result of educational differences or nursing specialties, which can result in expressions of horizontal violence. This tension of differences and unequal power relationships was also evident as the participants described their perceptions of the relationships between staff nurses and nurses in management positions. Each participant described experiences with nurses in management roles who have adopted marginal behaviors, who act like an oppressor, and who identify with the dominant culture of medicine and the health care bureaucracy, rather than with nursing. Most participants said that such oppressive action contributes to their feeling powered-over and unsupported by nurses in management positions. In the following narrative, Maude described the dynamics of the marginal identity and behaviors of nurses in management positions:

Maude: I mean our whole culture is that way. We're all brought up to believe there's somebody on top and somebody on the bottom and the only way to get on top is to act like the guy on top and climb over the people that are on the bottom. So, nursing is no different. There are a lot of rewards for the nurses that act that way; weekends off, you get to wear a lab coat, you get to decide what is going to happen on the floor. There are a lot of rewards . . .

Participants identified another tension in the relationships between staff nurses and nurses in management roles as originating in feelings of separateness, distance, or disconnection from staff nurses or nursing in general by some nurses in management roles. Monetary rewards and other quality-of-life distinctions were also described as contributing to feelings of separation and class distinctions between staff and nurse managers.

Regarding the term *horizontal violence*, some participants also presented an extremely valid critique. While they acknowledged that the expression does describe aspects of their lived experience, they also were concerned that the use of *horizontal* or *peer* from a narrow perspective could replicate unequal power relationships and hierarchies. Generally, however, the participants defined *horizontal* in an egalitarian sense. In this broad definition, horizontal violence was applied to all people who experience oppression in the world, including patients, women, and all nurses regardless of their position within an institution or society. In addition, participants critiqued the word *violence* as being a male-defined term that, if interpreted too literally, misses its more insidious expressions.

As voiced by the participants, descriptions of horizontal violence had to do with differences: differences in values, knowledge, education, role, sexuality, and the need to feel powerful. Participants described horizontal violence as a nursing reality that stems from oppression and oppressive conditions under which nurses try to make themselves feel better by disregarding the differences in others or by being unable to tolerate those differences.

Theme: Searching for ways to overcome oppression involves a personal and collective process of consciousness raising and transformation

It's a big cycle. Either you feed in to it or you try to break the chain—
Maude

In this last theme, participants described ways in which they tried to overcome the reality of oppression and how those efforts affected their relationships with one another and all aspects of their lives. Each participant described how the process of consciousness raising about oppression has helped to begin to transform their oppressive realities. Several participants named consciousness raising as a freeing experience.

The women also talked about how easy it was to continue to replicate unequal power relationships and horizontal violence either knowingly or unknowingly because of the environment. They spoke about how this way of living was so ingrained that we were not even consciously aware of all the ways we bought, and buy, into the oppression of others and even act it out ourselves. During the interviews and the group meeting, "false" consciousness or "blind spots" were uncovered and discussed as a tenacious and insidious experience. The following narratives provide examples of this experience:

Julia: *We feed right into it—get sucked in [without even knowing it]. You constantly have to separate your values from the institution.*

Margaret: *The class issue is very difficult for me . . . It never occurred to me [until hearing about it in this work]. I don't think about it at all, but listening to what other people have to say, now I'm understanding that I've been privileged. I ignore it so I don't believe it exists. But, obviously it does. I have opened my eyes about myself.*

It was very clear through the process of dialogue that the participants view personal and collective consciousness raising as integral in the empowerment of others. Maude describes the hopes and the potential for transformation through the empowerment of others:

Maude: *I think everyone is oppressed, not just women. The way society is structured, it takes away the impulse to reach out. When your consciousness is raised, suddenly it's not as easy to turn your back on someone. Then you reach out to them. . . . This applies to every part of your community. If you could reach out to . . . everyone you meet, suddenly the community would start to move in a different rhythm . . .*

Several participants told how the work environment makes a difference in their experience of oppression and horizontal violence. Several other participants described how both formal collaborative practice structures to improve relationships with physicians and supportive nurse managers can make a difference in how oppression is experienced.

Important here is the development of a sense of personal power as a means to overcome and transform oppressive realities. The development of personal power meant something different for each woman, but when viewed collectively, the paths they have chosen to develop this sense of self are remarkable. Their lists of ways for developing a sense of personal power include refusing to view self as a victim, honoring and living their values, learning about feminism and becoming women-identified, seeking knowledge as a path to excellence in nursing, keeping their focus on the patient, developing pride in nursing, and finding a safe place.

Most of the women described feminist thinking as a way for them to develop a sense of personal strength, resulting in refusal of the victim role. As Lillian asserted, "I am a hard person to power over." Participants acknowledged that as they have continued to learn more about feminist thinking, they are able to recognize, honor, and deeply value their woman-ness. As Maude said, "Every year I get a little older and things are beginning to click into place. I can move on and push some of the garbage aside."

Personal strength was also described as resulting from a clear sense of understanding personal values and honoring those values, as described in the following narrative:

> Charlotte: Well, I think when I distill it all out, it comes down to what is valued. Where is the value? What is it that motivates me to behave in a certain way? How am I authentic? And, if I am asked to act in an oppressive way or if I am asked to be a victim, neither makes me comfortable. And so I removed myself from the victim role, but I needed to develop skills to do that—and awareness. First I had to realize that I was acting as a victim and then I had to figure out how to get out of that role. And then [I had to figure out] how to live my values . . .

Many of the participants attributed their focus on patient care and pride in or identification with the culture of nursing as ways to develop their sense of personal strength. For Judy, this pride is her motivation for learning and developing clinical excellence:

> Judy: I really very much feel that I am a sincere person . . . I do. Like I'm not trying to be anything I'm not or trying to grasp upward to be a professional or anything else. I couldn't care less. But I do want to be excellent. I want to be extremely excellent. I want to understand things.

For Margaret, the development of self and personal sense of power involved finding a safe place where the experience of oppression is diminished:

> Margaret: I'm staying away from people that are horizontally violent and I'm working on ways to surround myself with people who I respect and have respect for me. I'm pulling away from hospital-type work right now because, I find in my particular situation, it's like a real ghetto for me . . . My peace is that I know I can pull away and find other ways to take care of myself.

This last theme is about the hope of transformation through empowering ourselves, raising our consciousness, becoming aware of our blind spots, and empowering others. The voices of the women who participated in this work are as unique and wonderful as each of them. The salient points about their individual experiences of oppression and their hopes and visions to overcome and transform this reality are the findings of this research. Collectively, their voices can inform nursing about the process of recovery and transformation.

Study Limitations

In this study, I attempted to describe the lived experience of the participants and the uniqueness of their reality. The lack of a greater understanding of the context or setting in which these women work prevents a certain thickness in the description of the narratives from which the themes emerged. Additionally, if the study had occurred within a specific context or group setting, the potential for a transformative or emancipatory process would have been perhaps more meaningful to the participants and the work itself.

The sample posed limitations as well. Dialogue with nurses outside the critical-care or acute-care setting may have raised different issues. Including the voices of women of color, nurses from other ethnic origins or cultures, and older nurses may have also resulted in a different set of descriptions about the oppression of nurses and experiences of horizontal violence.

Recommendations for future research include conducting a study using participatory, emancipatory methodology to explore specific context and allow for direct action as a result. Also, further studies about specific components of the named dimensions of oppression and horizontal violence would contribute greatly to understanding the dynamics of this problem.

DISCUSSION

Although the experiences of horizontal violence described by the women in this study are unique, they are not isolated. In a broad sense, the expression of horizontal violence is yet another dimension of the hegemony of domination in which powering-over others and the intolerance of differences is primary.

This perspective of the multiplicities of oppression has informed the development of an interactive model for understanding and overcoming oppression. As developed by Alperin (1990), the dimensions of the interactive model include the following concepts:

(1) There are many types of oppression; (2) A single form of oppression should not be considered a priori to be the driving force in all contexts;

(3) The different types of oppression interact with one another in complex ways; and (4) Eliminating a single form of oppression, even if it were the primary or original source of all other oppression, would not automatically eliminate all other forms of oppression (p. 27).

Proponents of the interactive model, such as Alperin (1990) and Bunch (1990), advocate that the elements of social diversity are positive and should be honored. However, they argue that within our present social system, there has been imposed upon these social differences a hierarchy of values that "is used to justify the lower status and discriminatory treatment of particular groups" (Alperin, p. 28).

The interactive model poses as strategies for the transformation of oppressive reality the processes of consciousness raising and developing alliances within individual groups and among diverse groups toward social justice through political action (Alperin, 1990; Bunch, 1990; Lorde, 1984; Pheterson, 1990). For nursing, the interactive model offers the hope that in the naming of the multiplicities of our oppression we will find the strength, through our connections with each other, to resist and transform such oppressions.

Using the concepts of consciousness raising in the interactive model described by Alperin (1990), nurses must first "shed any remnants of self-hatred" we have acquired as a result of our socialized oppression. To do this, we may first need to separate ourselves in a safe place to name ourselves, connect with each other, and rediscover our history. This process of identification is in itself a transformative step that requires a supportive environment—a safe place of our own design.

Yet, this is hardly enough. We also need to examine our personal and culturally ingrained blind spots, including critical appraisal of our own relationships with other nurses who may be different from us in some way. We need to honor and respect our differences within nursing while working toward eliminating the fragmentation and conflicts the differences can cause if we allow them to.

Additionally, we need to examine the unequal power relationships inherent in our current relationships and practices within nursing education, leadership, and management structures. We need to eliminate the elitist, marginal behaviors of nurses from their most overt to their more insidious expressions. This challenge is most enlightening when used as a template against nursing structures, practices, and leadership strategies created to "empower" nurses. With a raised consciousness about the multiple forms of oppression, nurses must critically evaluate and be clear about the motives behind "empowerment" models such as primary nursing, case management, clinical ladder systems, shared governance, collective bargaining, and educational entry level into practice.

Transformation involves not only an increased awareness of the multiplicities of oppression, but direct action toward a goal of freedom from domination for the oppressed and the oppressor (Freire, 1970). The building of alliances to bring about social change has been called feminist and nursing praxis (Chinn, 1989). Wheeler and Chinn (1984) defined praxis as the "thoughtful reflection and action that occurs in synchrony, in the direction of transforming the world" (p. 2). The concept of nursing praxis takes alliance building to the stage of political action. In nursing, social activism has been described as the ultimate expression of the ethic of caring in a health care system and society in the throes of severe crisis (MacPherson, 1989b; Moccia, 1988). The goal of social activism is creating a world of peace and pleasure.

In this study, I have discussed the project of naming the reality of the many dimensions of oppression in the world of nurses, including the horizontal violence which results from and replicates this oppressive reality. I have also discussed recovery and transformation through developing a new consciousness about oppression and building alliances toward a goal of social action or nursing praxis. The research findings are the voices of the women as they share their stories about their pain caused by oppression and their hopes and dreams for recovery and transformation.

The process of the work has been a personal journey. As the process began, I questioned my ability to maintain my nursing practice in the oppressive structure of the hospital setting. While I continued to hold onto my deep commitment to the value of my work as a nurse, the weight of oppression was heavy on my spirit. As a result of this work, I have come to a new way of knowing and affirmation for my commitment to nursing. I have uncovered blind spots about the oppressive characteristics and behaviors which I was imposing on others, and realize there are probably more blind spots that haven't yet revealed themselves to me. I feel I have now some specific patterns with which to weave alliances with other nurses and take action toward uncovering oppressive structures within nursing. Finally, I am no longer afraid of negative interpretations about bringing this aspect of nurses' relationships out into the open. As long as we are silent, the cycle of oppression will continue to separate us, cause us pain, and (dis)honor our diversity.

Recovery is the act of taking control over the forces that would destroy us. . . . Recovery is not an act that ignores the disease. Recovery is becoming stronger than the disease (Beth Brant, 1990, p. 118).

DISCUSSION QUESTIONS

1. In this paper, Skillings raises many questions about the internationalization of dominant culture in nursing. What is horizontal violence? How is this linked to oppressed group behavior?

2. What alternatives are suggested in this research for transforming distorted power relations in nursing? If an "interactive" model of oppressions is valid, what sorts of coalition or alliance building would this imply for nursing?

3. Comparing this paper with those of Turkoski, O'Neill, and Thompson, several questions are raised about the utility of continuing to rely on professional ideology as a mechanism for establishing political unity in nursing. Given these alternative analyses, what are some other sorts of political agenda(s) that might develop among and between different communities of nurses?

REFERENCES

Allen, D., Benner, P., & Diekelmann, N. (1986). Three paradigms for nursing research. In P. Chinn (Ed.), *Nursing research methodology*. Rockville, MD: Aspen Publishers.

Alperin, D. (1990). Social diversity and the necessity of alliances: Developing feminist perspective. In L. Albrecht & R. Brewer (Eds.), *Bridges of power: Women's multicultural alliances*. Philadelphia: New Society Publishers.

Ashley, J. (1973). This I believe: About power in nursing. *Nursing Outlook, 21*(1), 637–641.

Ashley, J. (1980). Power in structured misogyny: Implications for the politics of care. *Advances in Nursing Science, 2*(3), 3–21.

Brant, B. (1990). Recovery and transformation: The blue heron. In L. Albrecht & R. Brewer (Eds.), *Bridges of power: Women's multicultural alliances*. Philadelphia: New Society Publishers.

Bunch, C. (1990). Making common cause: Diversity and coalitions. In L. Albrecht & R. Brewer (Eds.), *Bridges of power: Women's multicultural alliances*. Philadelphia: New Society Publishers.

Chinn, P. (1989). Nursing patterns of knowing and feminist thought. *Nursing & Health Care, 10*(2), 70–75.

Chinn, P., & Wheeler, C. (1985). Feminism and nursing. *Nursing Outlook*, 33(2), 74–77.

Connors, D. (1988). A continuum of researcher-participant relationships: An analysis and critique. *Advances in Nursing Science*, 10(4), 32–42.

Fanon, F. (1963). *The wretched of the earth*. New York: Grove Press.

Freire, P. (1970). *The pedagogy of the oppressed*. New York: The Seabury Press.

French, M. (1985). *Beyond power*. New York: Summit Books.

Greenleaf, N. (1982). The politics of self-esteem. In E. Hein & J. Nicholson (Eds.), *Contemporary leadership behavior: Selected readings* (2nd ed). Boston: Little Brown.

Keen, P. (1988, June). *Caring for ourselves*. Paper presented at a conference of the Doctoral Student Group and Center for Human Caring. School of Nursing, University of Colorado, Denver, CO.

Lather, P. (1986). Research as praxis. *Harvard Educational Review*, 56(3), 257–277.

Lincoln, Y., & Guba, E. (1985). *Naturalistic Inquiry*. Beverly Hills, CA: Sage.

Lorde, A. (1984). Age, race, class and sex: Women redefining difference. In *Sister outsider: Essays and speeches*. Trumansburg, NY: The Crossing Press.

MacPherson, K. (1989a, June). *Looking at caring and nursing through a feminist lens*. Paper presented at a conference, Caring and Nursing: Explorations in feminist perspectives. University of Colorado Science Center, School of Nursing, Center for Human Caring, Denver, CO.

MacPherson, K. (1989b). A new perspective on nursing and caring in a corporate context. *Advances in Nursing Science*, 11(4), 32–39.

Maguire, P. (1987). *Doing participatory research: A feminist approach*. Amherst, MA: The Center for International Education, School of Education, University of Massachusetts.

Melosh, B. (1982). *The physician's hand*. Philadelphia: Temple University Press.

Moccia, P. (1988). At the faultline: Social activism and caring. *Nursing Outlook*, 36(1), 30–33.

Mullen, J. (1987, March). *Violent/nonviolent nursing behaviors: Toward a new theory of consciousness*. Paper presented at a conference, Violence Against Women, University of Massachusetts at Amherst.

Oakley, A. (1988). Interviewing women: A contradiction in terms. In H. Roberts (Ed.), *Doing feminist research*. New York: Routledge.

Pheterson, G. (1990). Alliances between women: Overcoming internalized oppression and internalized domination. In L. Albrecht & R. Brewer (Eds.), *Bridges of power: Women's multicultural alliances*. Philadelphia: New Society Publishers.

Reverby, S. (1987). A caring dilemma: Womanhood and nursing in historical perspective. *Nursing Research, 36*(1), 6–11.

Reverby, S. (1989). *Ordered to care.* Cambridge: Cambridge University Press.

Roberts, S. (1983). Oppressed group behavior: Implications for nursing. *Advances in Nursing Science, 5*(4), 21–30.

Schroyer, T. (1973). *The critique of domination.* New York: George Braziller.

Skillings, L. (1990). *Perceptions and feelings of nurses about horizontal violence as an expression of oppressed group behavior.* Masters thesis, University of Southern Maine School of Nursing, Portland, ME.

Stevens, P. (1989). A critical social reconceptualization of environment in nursing: Implications for methodology. *Advances in Nursing Science, 11*(4), 56–58.

Thompson, J. (1987). Critical scholarship: The critique of domination in nursing. *Advances in Nursing Science, 10*(1), 27–38.

Thompson, J. (1990). Hermeneutic inquiry. In L. Moody (Ed.), *Advancing nursing science through research.* Newbury Park, CA: Sage.

Wheeler, C. & Chinn, P. (1984). *Peace and power: A handbook of feminist process.* Buffalo: Margaretdaughters, Inc.

Index

Abel, E., 72
Adler, A., 119
African Americans
    "black" designation and ethnicity/
        social class theories, 41–44
    identity politics, 27–28
    Tuskeegee syphilis experiment, 5,
        47–48
Allen, D., 141, 171
Allen, J., 85
Alperin, D., 180–181
American Nurses Association (ANA),
    143
Anzaldua, Z., 31
Aristotle, 70–71
Ashley, J., 109, 170

Bales, R. F., 57
Banks-Wallace, Jo Ann, 45
Barrow, E., 134
Baumgart, A. J., 141

Belenky, M., 88
Bell, S., 104–105
Benhabib, S., 8, 71, 78
Benner, P., 11, 171
Beyond Power, 168, 171
Bleier, R., 7
Bogaert, A. F., 46–47
Botha, M. E., 130
Bradshaw, J., 85–86
Brodribb, S., 109
Brody, E. M.
    Women in the Middle, 56
Bunch, C., 181
Burfoot, A., 109–110
Bushy, A., 108
Butterfield, P. G., 64
Buxton, Peter, 48

Canadian Research Institute for the
    Advancement of Women
    (CRIAW), 98, 101

Card, C., 76, 77
Caregiving and ethics for nursing,
    69–81
  feminist philosophy, 77–79
  gender, historical influence of,
    70–71
  interpersonal caring, models of,
    73–75
  labor, division of, 72–73
  Noddings, feminist critique of,
    75–77
Caregiving, feminist critique of
    Watson, 85–95
  reflections of author, 92–95
  theory in general, 87–89
  transpersonal/spiritual focus of,
    90–92
  ungenderedness of, 89–90
Caregiving from feminist perspective,
    53–64
  alpha and beta biases, 56–57
  boundaries, work and family
    spheres, 60
  definition and ubiquity of, 55
  ethnocentric/andocentric bias,
    62–63
  ideology of, 55–56
  invisible work aspect, 60–62
  private vs. public spheres, effects
    of separation, 59
  private vs. public spheres,
    historical perspective, 58
  socialization of women, 57
  value of household production,
    58–59
  women as natural caregivers, 56
  women, influx to workplace of,
    59–60
Chapman, C. M., 134
Chesler, P., 117
Chinn, P., 92, 170–171
  Peace and Power, 173, 182
Chodorow, N., 57, 75, 122–123,
    124–125
Chrisman, N. J., 36, 49

Clark, M., 134
Classism, 140
Colliere, M. F., 60
Conners, D., 172
Corea, G., 102
"Culture Care Diversity" (Leininger),
    55

Daly, M., 85, 91
de Lauretis, T., 43
DeMark, J., 85
Diekelmann, N., 171
"Dyke Methods," 86

Eisenstein, Z., 152
Elshtain, J., 70–71
Equal Rights Amendment (ERA), 13,
    143, 163
Erikson, E., 120
Erikson, E. H., 57
Essentialism, 27–31
Eugenics in name of science/health,
    45–46

Fanon, F., 169
Feminism
  caregiving and, 53–64, 69–81,
    85–95
  gender identity and, 122–126
  horizontal violence/oppressed
    group behavior, 167–182
  identity politics and essentialism,
    25–31
  nursing, ethics for, 69–81
  nursing process and social
    construction, 132–135
  nursing, professionalism in,
    137–145, 149–164
  reproductive health care and,
    97–111
  science, philosophy of, 1–13
  and theory, use of, 87–89, 93–94
Feminist Theory and Philosophies of
    Man, 93
Field, M., 107

Fields, B., 42–43
Firestone, Shulasmith, 101
Fisher, B., 72
Flax, J., 122, 124–125
Flexner report, 138, 139, 142
Folan, M., 130
Foucault, M., 37, 102
Frank, D., 105
Freire, P., 169–170, 171
French, M.
    Beyond Power, 168, 171
Freud, S., 118–119
Frye, M., 85

Gadow, S., 73–74
Gallagher, J., 106–107
Gay community, identity politics and
    essentialism, 25–31
Gender
    absence in Watson's theory,
        89–90
    caregiving and, 53–64, 69–81,
        85–95
    professionalism and gender
        analysis, 144–145
Gender identity, female and women's
        health, 117–126
    concept, historical development,
        118–122
    feminist views on, 122–125
    nursing perspective, feminist,
        125–126
Gibeau, J., 61
Gidden, A., 9–13
Gilchrist, J. M., 141
Gilligan, C., 57, 74–75, 78, 122
Giroux, H., 31–32
Goldmark report, 139, 141–142
Gordon, D. R., 40
Gross, E., 27–28
Guillaumine, C., 43

Habermas, J., 5–6, 132–133, 134, 152
Hagan, K., 85
Hampson, J. G., 120, 121

Hampson, J. L., 120, 121
Hanmer, J., 103, 109
Haraway, D., 38
Harding, S., 2, 4
Hare-Mustin, R. T., 54, 56–57,
        58–59
Hekman, S., 27
Hoagland, S., 75
"Home", constructions of in identity
        politics, 25–28, 31–33
hooks, b., 85, 140, 141
    Talking Back, 87–88
Hooyman, N. R., 61–62
Horizontal violence and oppressed
        group behavior, 167–182
    critical social/feminist theory, 171
    domination, 169–170
    literature review, 169–172
    nursing, oppressed group behavior
        in, 170–171, 173–182
    research study, methodology of,
        168, 172–173
Horney, K., 119–120
Houston, B., 75–76, 77

Identity politics, 21–33
    essentialism in non-nursing
        communities, 27–31
    "home" constructions, 25–28,
        31–33
    nursing and, 24–27
    nursing education and critical
        pedagogy, 31–33

Johnson, S., 85
Jones, E., 119–120
Jones, J. H., 48

Kestenberg, J., 120
Klein, R., 102–103
Kleinman, Arthur, 36
Kobart, L., 130
Koch, L., 100, 102
Kolder, V., 106–107

Kroll, D., 108
Kuhn, T., 4, 6

Lamar, E., 105
Language and reification of nursing
	care, 129–135
	ethics of practice, concealed or
		revealed, 131
	nursing practice, social
		construction of, 132–135
	nursing process, 130–131
Lather, P., 9, 85, 172, 173
Leininger, M. M., 36, 55
Lesbianism
	identity politics and essentialism,
		25–31
	oppression and horizontal
		violence, 175
Leslie, C., 46
Levine, M. E., 131
Lifton, R. J., 45–46
Lorde, A., 169
Lugones, M., 87
Lundh, U., 132, 133
Lundy, C., 117

MacKinnon, C., 123–125
Maguire, P., 172
Manitoba Association of Registered
	Nurses, 143
Manitoba Organization of Nurses
	Association, 143
Marmaduke, A., 104–105
Matt, B., 108
Mayeroff, M., 87, 90
Melosh, B., 170
Miller, A., 85, 93
Miller, J. B., 122
Milne, B., 105
Moccia, P., 149
Money, J., 120, 121
Morgall, J., 100, 102
Moss, K., 100, 102
Mullen, J., 170

National Association of Colored
	Graduate Nurses (NACGN),
	142–143
National Black Nurses Association
	(NBNA), 142
National League for Nursing, 143
Native Americans. See Swinomish
	Tribe
Nelson, M., 72
Nietzsche, F., 93
Nightingale, Florence, 140
Noddings, N., 73, 75–77
Nursing: Human Science and Human
	Care, 89
Nye, A., 91
	Feminist Theory and Philosophies of
		Man, 93

Oakley, A., 172
O'Brien, M., 101, 109–110
Obstetrical intervention, court
		ordered, 105–111. See also
		Reproductive technology
	control of women, 106–107
	feminist/critical approach for
		nurses, lack of, 108–111
Omi, M., 41–42
Ontario Law Reform Commission
	Report on Human Artificial
		Reproduction and Related
		Matters, 100
Oppressed group behavior. See
		Horizontal violence and
		oppressed group behavior
Oregon Federation for Nursing, 143
Ovesey, L., 121

Pace-Owens, S., 105
Paige, K., 117
Parsons, M., 106–107
Parsons, T., 57
Peace and Power, 173, 182
Person, E., 121
Phillips, L. A., 63–64
Polednak, A. P., 38

Pope, D., 56
Popkewitz, T., 150
Poteet, G., 105
Pratt, M. B., 23
Professionalism in nursing, 137–145,
    149–164
    altruism and service, association
        with, 157–160
    classism, 140–141, 161–162
    critical analysis of, 149–164
    dress as symbol of, 160–161
    elite view of activism, 163
    genderism, 144, 162
    hierarchy and status, language of,
        154–156
    historical overview, 138–139
    ideology, 151–152, 153 fig.
    market protection, 156–157
    models, progressive, 142–144
    racism, 141–142, 162
    working class profession, 144–145

Quinn, N., 56

Race
    discourses on, 36–39
    ethnicity/class-based theories on,
        41–42
    ideologies of, 42–43
Race and health
    naturalism, 40–41
    research, problems in, 44–50
    silences, 36–37, 50
Randell, P., 108
Reagon, B., 32
Rempusheski, V. F., 63–64
*Report on Human Artificial Reproduction
    and Related Matters*, 100
Reproductive technology, 97–105,
    108–111. *See also* Obstetrical
    intervention, court ordered
    cost concern, 101
    critical woman-centered analysis
        for nursing, 108–110
    ethical and legal issues, 100

feminist concerns, 102–104
feminist/critical approach for
    nurses, lack of, 98–99,
    104–105, 110–111
social implications, 100
social roles and control of,
    100–101
Reverby, S., 170
Rew, L., 134
Rhodes, A. M., 108
Ricoeur, P., 129, 132
Riley, D., 70
Roberts, S., 167, 170
Rothman, B., 103
Rowland, R., 102–103
Rushton, J. P., 2, 46–47
Ryan, R., 61, 63

Sams, Lauranne, 142
Sandelowski, M., 105, 108, 110
Saran, Ama, 45
Schroyer, T., 171
Science, feminist philosophy of,
    1–13
    evidence/process, 2, 3, 4–9
    explanation, 2, 3, 9–13
    Gidden's theory of structuration,
        9–13
    ideology, problem of, 3–4
    relativism, 1–2, 8–9
    situatedness, 7–8
Scott, Joseph, 42
Seidman, S., 29–31
Sexual preference
    identity politics and, 25–31
    oppression and, 169
Sise, C. B., 108
Soder, M., 132, 133
Spallone, P., 102
    Warnock Report, The, 100,
        101–102
Spellman, E., 27, 87
Stevens, P., 171
Stoller, R., 120, 121
Swinomish Tribe, 49

Talking Back, 87–88
Taussig, M., 48
Theory and its uses, 87–89, 93–94
    escaping physicality and
        emotional needs, 93
Thompson, C., 119
Thompson, J., 151–152, 171, 172,
    173
Thompson, J. L., 9
Trebilcot, J., 86
    "Dyke Methods," 86
Tronto, J., 72
Tuskeegee syphilis experiment,
    47–48
Twomey, J. G., 108

Waerness, K., 132, 133
Walker, M., 78–79
Ward, D. H., 60
Warnock Report, The, 100, 101–102
Warren, M. A., 101, 102, 103
Watson, J., 74, 108–109, 131
    feminist critique of, 85–95
    Nursing: Human Science and
        Human Care, 89
Wheeler, C., 170–171
    Peace and Power, 173, 182
Williams, L., 100, 102, 103
Winant, H., 41–42
Women in the Middle, 56
Wyer, M., 56

Yamato, G., 41